# Life with Multiple Sclerosis

## Brian Groenenstein

# Dedication

This book is dedicated to my loving children Micaela Lee-Ann and Grant Groenenstein.

Also a special thanks to Claudette Ann Groenenstein, my mother, whose input has been tremendously helpful.

Also a special thanks to Celicia Selma Groenenstein and Tanya Lynne Piper

**Cover Design Grant Groenenstein**

**Copyright ©Brian Groenenstein**

# Prologue

When I was a young man in the prime of my adult life, I had neither worries nor cares; healthy, happy and thoroughly contented; invincibly infused with my daily life. This was my life, wild exciting and full of living. Like any young man of that age I was, for the worse part a rebel without a cause. My nights used to be wild and filled with fun and yes to a certain extent, some danger. But this was my life and the way I lived it. Along the way I had my share of enemies and friends. It was never easy to find balance in my life. There were tough times and also good times, but for the better part I have lived.

Little did I know that silently within this "vessel" that supports my life, an "enemy" was lurking in the shadows. This "vessel" - my body and brain that supports my ideas, my thoughts, my actions, my movements and for the most of it my life, one day decided to formulate a war on me. I did however notice the subtle warnings and hints that my "vessel" was signalling to me, but I had decided it would be for the best to ignore them. Regrettably because of my stupid neglect of said warnings the "enemy" within me pounced.

From then on nothing would ever be the same, and this "enemy" had a name: Multiple Sclerosis. This "enemy" decided to slowly rob me of my ideas, my thoughts, my actions, my movements and yes; my life. For the next 3 years it bombarded me with one relentless attack after the other, not allowing me to fight back. This enemy was far bigger than me and I was fighting a losing battle. But just as suddenly as this war was declared a cease fire broke out. And I thought that I might have won the war, as everything turned to normality. But normal from then on would never be the same, as the battle scars were there. My casualty list was nerve damage to the right side of my face and visual damage to my eyes. Ever the optimist I decided to make the best of this, as I thought the battle was won, but MS had not retreated, but only withdrawn to regroup.

Always apprehensive of this "enemy", I decided to carry on living, but so did my "enemy". It left me in peace and for the next couple of years, I was content and so I thought was my "enemy" within. After a good couple of years I now could call myself one of those that have survived Multiple Sclerosis, but as with any good "enemy" it was re-evaluating its battle plan. Just as suddenly as the first attacks, it launched another offensive on me, but this time with different tactics and more intensive. However this time I was ready for it, and I fought back with all my ability. My enemy now had the strongest opposition ever, as I was armed with an arsenal of information on MS, and I too had changed my tactics. I altered my way of living, to a healthier way of life. We are now locked into a constant battle, but this knowledge and lifestyle has equipped me with the upper hand, and I am for the better part able to win all these battles, and perhaps one day I will win this war. For the most part I viewed my "enemy" as "friend" in a cold war and refused to be blindsided by it. I can respect all its manoeuvres, but will block them with all my knowledge and fortitude I can gather. Multiple Sclerosis knows me and I know it, and my clear message to MS is:" I might have MS but MS will never have me". Multiple Sclerosis is now a part of me, and we share the same "vessel", and to a certain extent it defines who I am today.

This is my message to all my fellow MS patients: never give in, and never surrender. You are the stronger one and coupled with your will and knowledge it will help you in win this battle. Arm yourself with knowledge of MS and know the signs of an attack. Listen to your body and live a healthy and balanced life and rest when your body tells you to. With every battle that you win, you will eventually win the war. And one day we will triumph over this "enemy and friend". That day will go down in the history of MS as our victory...

Stay strong and keep moving, and live your life to the best of your abilities

# My journey with Multiple Sclerosis

The last two years was probably the hardest years of my life. I have become the skeleton of the man I used to be. How did I get here is the big question, and what transpired to get me where I am today, and where am I going?
To know where you are going, you need to realize where you came from in the first place. Take a step backwards and look at your own life, only then will you be able to see where you came from and what the future has in store for you.

Today I am nearly 50 years old, and in a place where I don't particularly want to be. I have lost all in life, the persons I loved and nearly everything I've owned. I barely survived the last 5 years of my life, and at times I was ready to give up all hope of any normality. I am now standing back and reflecting on my life, to see where I came from.

In 1993 I was involved in a minor accident on a motor way. Driving home from work one night I realized something was wrong with my eyesight. A couple of days earlier I had started to get blurred vision and terrible headaches. (I must add that as a teenager, I had an eye injury and complication from the injury left me with only partial sight in my right eye). Thinking that this was only the after effects of the flu I had a week before, I did not pay much attention to it. But on this particular night something was different. My eyesight started blurring very badly and I could hardly see, and I misjudged the distance to the vehicle in front of me. Slamming on the brakes I realized it was too late, and I rear ended the car in front of me.

I was taken to the local hospital with some minor injuries, but what was lurking beneath the surface was far more damaging. It was not an injury, but a particular symptom that became a known problem and also an indicator of things to come in my life.

What followed next was a series of events that I would never forget in my entire life.

The local intern, a student doctor who examined me, had just completed a rotation in the neurology wing of a big hospital. And after asking a couple of question, he decided to take a bit more of an interest in my underlying symptoms and rather let the small cut and bump on my head take a backseat. He was more intrigued by the flu and the blurred vision. This was also the first time that my path crossed with the small hammer, which has also become a too familiar part of my life. After prodding away with the hammer, and a couple of pin pricks, and some test on my now nearly totally blinded eyes, a decision was made. I was told that he would rather transfer me to the neurological wing of Tygerberg hospital, as he suspected that underlying symptoms was part of a bigger picture.

The next three weeks was a very interesting part of my life. I woke up in Tygerberg hospital, drugged to the eyeballs to relieve excruciating pain.  The blurred vision from the night before had nearly completely blinded me and was now also very painful. I stumbled out of bed with very limited vision, and was also looking for relief of another problem. I needed a nicotine fix urgently, and upon asking for direction, I was guided by a nurse to the smoking lounge.

Back in the ward, in came the hammer squad, as I now refer to them. Back in bed, a couple of students arrived with their chief and leader, the neurologist. Again the hammer prodding started, and the needle pricking followed. Along with that were the constant eye reflex testing and the shining of a small bright light into my already painful eyes. About an hour later they left, still leaving me hanging as to what was wrong with me. I was hammered, scratched and pricked, but still no answer from the leader and chief. The only answer to my questions was, "We will get to the bottom of this, and we just needed to do more tests".

Later on lunch came, the normal awful tasting hospital food and a couple of blind strolls back and forth, from my ward feeling my way to the smoking lounge. More drugs followed, and later I was whisked off for what was to be my first encounter with the Sensory Evoke Potential (SEP) test.  Sitting on this contraption, the mini version of the electric chair, with a couple of leads and probes on my head, I was connected to a computerised machine. The drugs having now worn off, I was not allowed any pain medication until this test was done.

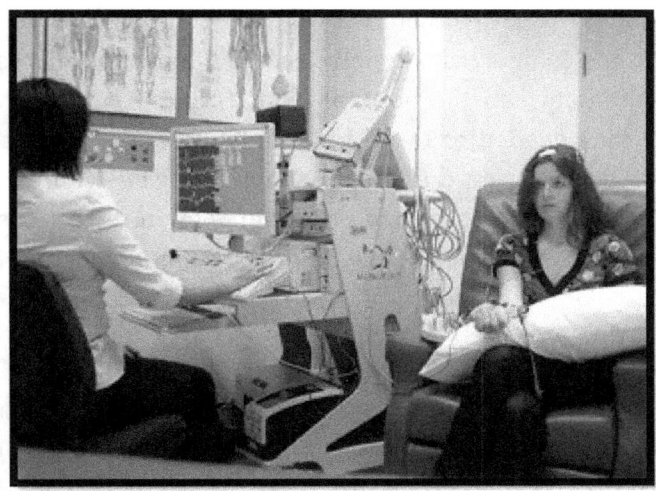

[1] Sensory Evoke Potential Test. (Image courtesy of Dr Karl Ng)

A little elaboration will be needed on this specific test for the uninformed. A Sensory Evoke Potential test consists of a couple of ECG probes placed on the scalp, neck and sometimes on your back, in strategic places. Then certain probes get attached to your arms and legs normally at the wrist and ankles. Then, small electrical impulses are passed through the probes on your wrist or ankle. The test itself is not painful, but will cause certain muscle and fingers and toes to twitch or jerk from small electrical shocks. This test measures the impulse from the limb up to the time the brain responds to it. In effect, it tests the reaction time of your nerves and brain to respond to a particular stimulus, and in this case, the small electrical shocks. This test has been in use in modern medication since the 1970, although these days is far more sophisticated than in the 1970, thanks to the invention of modern science and the computer.

After about an hour and a half, the test was done and I was sent packing back to my hospital bed, but still with no answer. By then it was time for another shot of pain medication and a couple of nicotine fixes. The big chief arrived with one or two hammer squad students, looked at my chart and some of the results, then informed me that they will need to get a couple more test done and I should try to relax. My first thought was relax, "Tell me how you do that from going from flu to near total blindness in two weeks. I would certainly love to see how they get that right". Luckily the drugs kept me from uttering these words out loud.

The first familiar voices that night was of my then first wife and her girlfriend who came to visit me, and brought me some much needed cigarettes and some snacks which were be a welcome alternative to the hospital food. The visit was much appreciated considering that they needed to travel for nearly an hour there and back. Questions followed, but I was in no position to supply my wife with any answers, as I had none to give.  Another night followed and yet another mysterious symptom also appeared. My right side of my body were slowly going numb, and I noticed a slight limp when I walked to the smoking lounge.

Early next morning after breakfast the big chief again arrived, with his entourage of white coated interns. Another session of hammer blows and some more testing, including the scratching of the bottom of my feet with a pencil and watching which way my toes curled. All I heard were the words that I have a positive Babinski reflex. Only later on in life did I learn the meaning of these words, this only after my own research, as the men in white tend to talk about you, but not to you. Probably in their minds, these words will have no meaning to you, and since you are on a need to know basis, it seems pointless explaining it to you as you do not need to know this.

Well I am going to explain to you, the reader, as this is something you need to know. Doctors tend to think of patients as unintellectual beings that could not understand these complex terms.

A Positive Babinski reflex in a new born is normal, however from the age of two years it is not normal. In healthy new born babies, toes will pull up and fan out on a positive reflex, as the nerves to the brain from the spinal cord are not fully developed. In neurology in adults this is a sign of some serious brain trauma, or an indicator of some form of nerve damage. In a healthy Babinskis Reflex the toes will curl downwards and curl in. I had a positive Babinskis reflex, and looking back today I am glad that the men in white did not educate me as to what this means. At least I did not worry about my toes not going in the right direction.

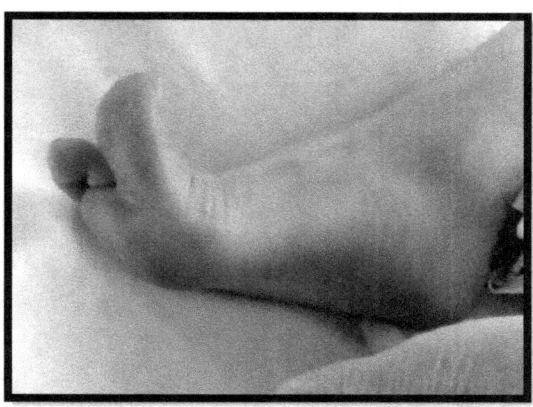

[2] Positive Babinskis Reflex

That afternoon I was again whisked away for another test. This time it was the Visual Evoke Potential (VEP) test. The VEP test is similar to SEP but with a slight difference, and at least no involvement of electrical shocks. Similar probes get placed on the scalp, but a lot more than in a SEP, or at least that is how I experienced it. You are then asked to watch a series of square patterns on a screen, being flashed at you. The speed and size differs, and one eye is tested at a time. The response time of the optic nerve to the brain's visual cortex is measured by some fancy piece of computer equipment. This response time is an indicator as to how the brain's visual cortex and optical nerve respond to light stimulus, and a slowed reaction is an indicator of some form of nerve or brain damage. This test is highly sensitive and can be an indicator of certain conditions, and is far more reliant than the testing of pupil reaction to light. Although in my case, my pupil reaction to light was clearly visible under normal light reaction testing. My right eye clearly responded differently than my left eye.

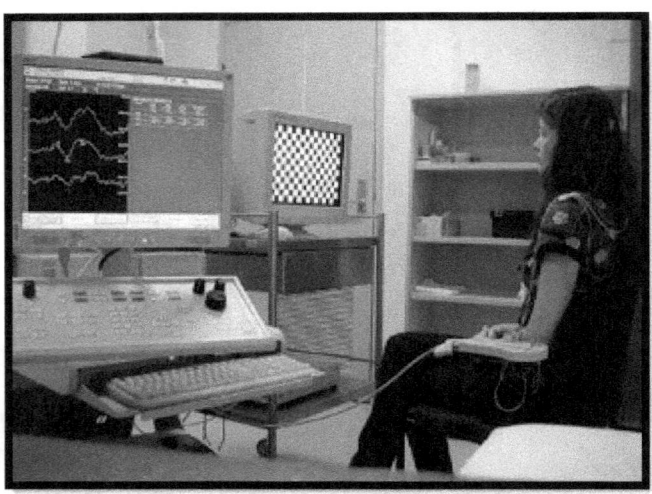

[3] Visual Evoke Potential test. (Image courtesy of Dr Karl Ng)

Again an hour or so later the test was done, and I could get much needed relief for my nicotine addiction and also some pain medication as well. I was denied any pain medication that morning again as it could interfere with the afternoon's test.

Very late that afternoon, I was set to have the first very uncomfortable test since my stay in hospital. The big chief arrived with a couple of nurses and again I was whisked through the door opposite to my ward. I was informed that I was about to receive a lumbar puncture. Now I have heard of this before in my life, and this got me very nervous. The Spinal Tap as it is commonly referred to as, is a very uncomfortable and can be traumatic for some patients.

Essentially, since you have no blood in your brain and something needs to feed your brain with the necessary oxygen, proteins etc. This is where CSF or Cerebral Spinal Fluid comes into play. CSF is the fluid that feeds your brain, and it is floating in this. The fluid contains glucose, proteins, and other substances that are also found in the blood. It is an essential test in all matters medical involving the brain including Multiple Sclerosis.

The dreaded spinal tap consist firstly of the numbing by local anaesthesia of the lower portion of your back normally just at about the pants line. Then a needle with a tap is inserted into the spinal cord between two vertebrae's. Spinal fluid is then extracted from the back and sent off for testing. The Spinal Fluid is normally clear, but in certain condition can have a darkish colour.

Spinal fluid that indicates a large number of immunoglobulin's or antibodies, as well as Oligoclonal bands or certain proteins that are the breakdown products of myelin is suggestive of MS. Immunoglobulin (Ig), is a large Y-shaped protein produced by B-cells that is used by the immune system to identify and neutralize foreign objects such as bacteria and viruses. Oligoclonal bands are bands of immunoglobulin. These findings indicate an abnormal autoimmune response within the brain and spinal cord, meaning that the body is attacking itself.

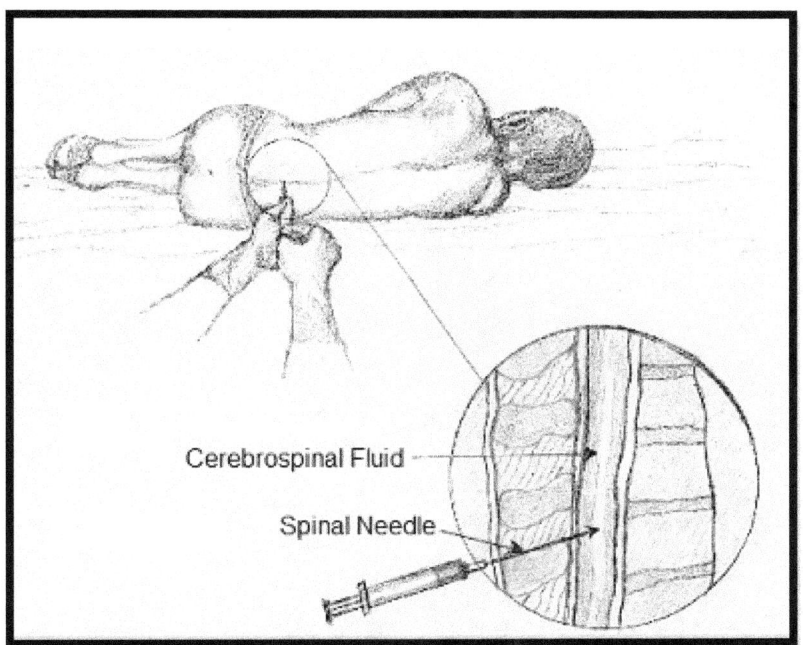

[4] Lumber Punch or spinal tap (Image courtesy of Claudette Ann Groenenstein)

90% of all patients with Multiple Sclerosis have Oligoclonal bands in their CSF. Increased immunoglobulin in the CSF and Oligoclonal bands are seen in many other brain and spinal cord conditions, but are very useful for diagnosing Multiple Sclerosis. As for the other 10% of MS patients that do not show up with these bands or antibodies, it does not rule out MS. Negative spinal taps have been noted in multiple sclerosis, and diagnoses is normally based on a larger picture like the magnetic resonance imaging (MRI), potential evoked tests and other neurological indicators.

Back in the ward the golden rule is to lay flat for at least a couple of hours after a spinal tap. But about an hour later I went for a much needed cigarette. Not heeding the doctors warning that it may be wise to lay flat as you may suffer from a terrible headache, I was now feeling the effects of this.

Night came and went like the day before, with some welcome visitors from the day before and a flower basket with chocolates from my employer. My eyesight had still not improved and the limp and numbness was still ever present. To a certain extend this became very worrying as it has been the third night since the accident and still I was no closer to getting any answers.

The usual morning routine with the men in white followed, and I was booked for a Magnetic Resonance Imaging (MRI) test and another test in the afternoon.

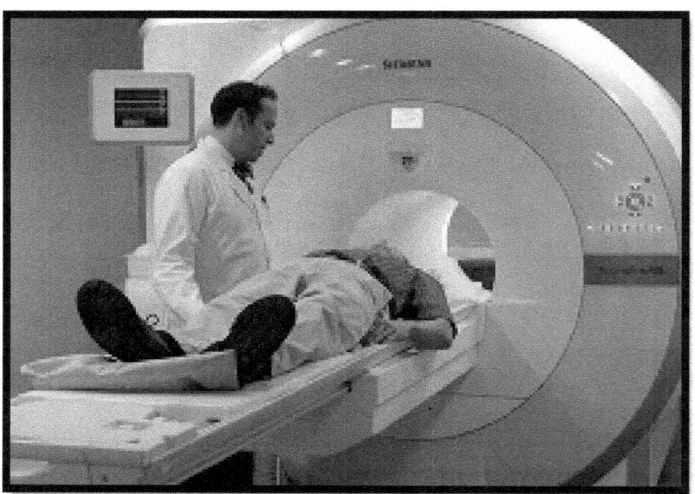

[5] Magnetic Resonance Imaging Test (Image courtesy of National Institute of Health (NIH))

Now I need to explain the function of the MRI to laymen, and the intriguing workings thereof. An MRI scan consists of a series of magnetic resonance images taken from the brain and spinal cord as in my case, but is also used to image the rest of the body's complicated setup and detail. In the 1950 this type of imaging was not available and good old x-rays were the only ones in use. An MRI consists of a powerful series of magnetic fields being used to align and spin the protons that are found in the makeup of the human body. Different radio frequencies spin these protons in different alignment to image the body, brain and spinal cord. These protons are basically found in the water of the human body, and since we consist of a large amount of water hence a large amount of protons. Protons are atomic particles found in the human body. A radio frequency current is briefly turned on, producing a varying electromagnetic field. This electromagnetic field has just the right frequency, known as the resonance frequency, to be absorbed and flip the spin of the protons in the magnetic field. After the electromagnetic field is turned off, the spins of the protons return to thermodynamic equilibrium and the bulk magnetization becomes re-aligned with the static magnetic field. During this relaxation, a radio frequency signal (electromagnetic radiation in the RF range) is generated, which can be measured with receiver coils. Hence it was give a name Magnetic Resonance Imaging or MRI for short. This Technology helps us see a very clear detail image of the brain, spinal cord and the rest of the human body.

Now to get into one of these massive machines, you need one precaution first, remove all metal objects on you as these have very powerful magnetic fields. Once inside you will probably get a little claustrophobic, as the tunnel is very narrow, and the noise it emanates can scare the pants off many a patient, even with the drug they give you beforehand to settle the nervousness. The whole scanning process takes about 1 hour or longer if they scan the brain and spinal cord. But we end up with a nice set of pictures like the one below, clearing showing the inner brain sliced in many pieces. Lovely piece of equipment; this MRI that sounds like a high speed washing machine with a couple of broken ball bearings, causing this racket inside.

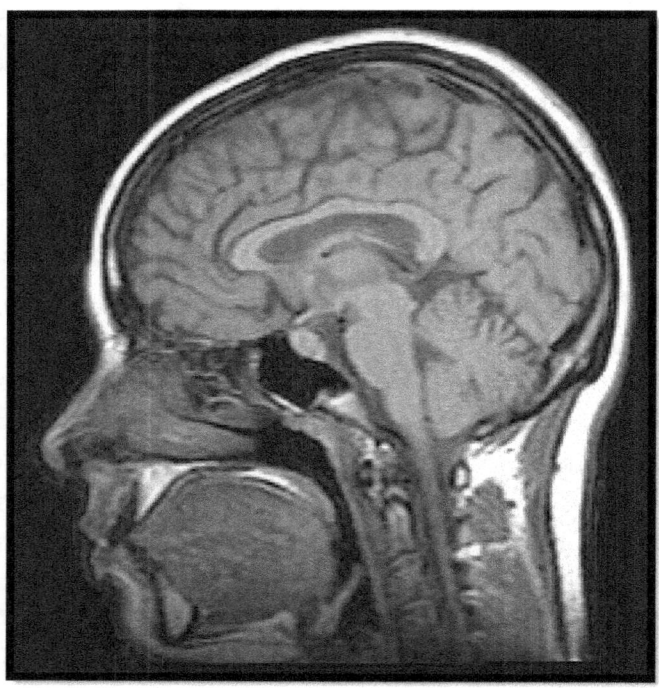

[6] MRI Image (Image source: Wikipedia)

Surviving this, I set off for my nicotine fix. Shortly there afterwards there was also a trip to have a Brainstem Auditory Evoked Potentials (BAEPs), a test to determine if there is any hearing function loss. This test is similar to the VEP, the difference being the auditory nerve is tested. Sensor probes are attached to the scalp, and a small clicking sound is played to the ear, by means of a headset or earplugs. A fancy piece of computer equipment measures the response time along the Auditory nerve to the brainstem. A delay in response is a clear indication of certain neural pathway damage.

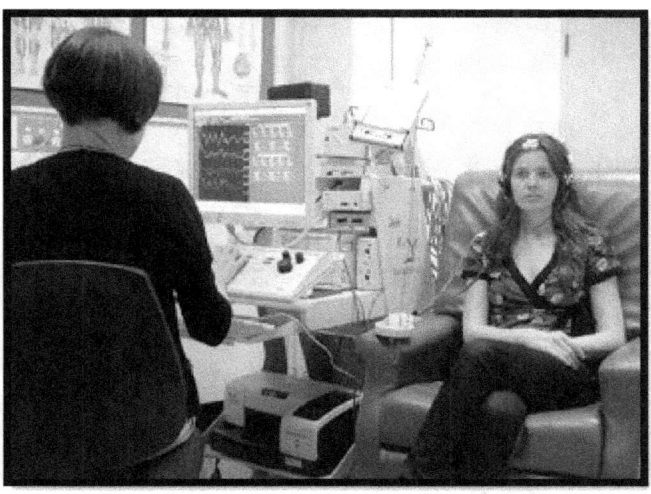

[7] Brainstem Auditory Evoked Potentials. (Image courtesy of Dr Karl Ng)

About three o'clock that afternoon the big chief and his crew arrived again, luckily for me this was the last time I was left without any answer. Although the answer was not at all anything I could have thought of it still shocked me to the core of my being. In the answering my question of "What is wrong with me?" without any great fanfare or sparing of my feelings, I was told I have Multiple Sclerosis.

What followed was a dialogue that to me was simply beyond my comprehension. I had a couple of thousands of questions running through my head, but the first one that popped into my mind was "Is this multiple whatever treatable?" I did not expect to receive the answer of "No".  Now anyone who has experienced a rapid onset of sudden vision loss and numbness on the right side the next question seems perfectly normal. "What is my prognosis and what am I to expect?"

Again another answer followed that stunned and shocked me, not believing what I was told for quite a while. If ever I need a cigarette or drugs it was right now. As far as treatment is concerned there is none, to heal it, but we could slow down the progression of this disease with the name of Multiple Sclerosis. I was to receive my first dose of medicine that afternoon already without any hesitation. And along came my first introduction to the intravenous steroid drip. As for my prognosis it was very hard to tell with exact certainty what would happen to me.

**Optical Coherence Tomography (OCT),** is a simple, non-invasive eye test which could offer a way to measure how fast Multiple Sclerosis is progressing in a patient. The test takes just a few minutes per eye and can be performed at an Ophthalmologist surgery. This test was introduced in 1993 to assists doctors in the examination of patients with serious diseases of the retina.

 When I was first diagnosed this test was not available at the hospital I was treated at, but is since being used in Multiple Sclerosis monitoring. I have had two OCT scans already and they clearly indicate a thinning of the retina.

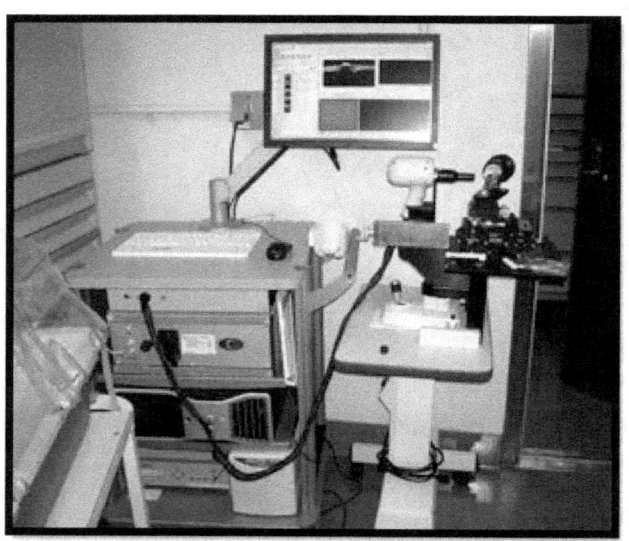

[8] Optical Coherence Tomography (Image Courtesy: National Eye Institute, National Institutes of Health (NEI/NIH).)

Optical Coherence Tomography is effectively an optical ultrasound, imaging reflections from within tissue to provide cross-sectional images.   The test determines the thickness of the retina. Retinal thinning is natural during the ageing process.

In a recent study carried out by John Hopkins University, they performed scans on 164 Multiple Sclerosis patients, measuring the thickness of the retina at the back of the eye. Their findings determined that patients with thinning of the retina had both earlier and more active forms of the disease. The patients received examination every six months for 21 months. They were also given a MRI brain scan once a year.

Monitoring Multiple Sclerosis is difficult because its course and symptoms can vary greatly from patient to patient. Researchers believe OCT could provide a good way to measure the progression and severity of the disease.

"As more therapies are developed to slow the progression of MS, testing retinal thinning in the eyes may be helpful in evaluating how effective those therapies are," the study researcher Dr Peter Calabresi said.

The results of the study concluded that the patients with relapses have about 42% increased thinning of the retina, than those that had no flare up or relapses. Also evident from MRI scan results show that in patients who had signs of active inflammation, indicated by gadolinium-enhancing lesions, the retina was thinning 54% faster. Patients whose disability was worsening during the study experienced 37% more thinning than those who had no changes in disability level.

The study was supported by the National Multiple Sclerosis Society, the National Eye Institute and Braxton Debbie Angela Dillon and Skip Donor Advisor Fund.

# The History of Multiple Sclerosis

**The Historical cases of Multiple Sclerosis Patients**
Multiple Sclerosis was first added to the medical books in 1868 by a French neurologist Jean-Martin Charcot. Before that there were some documented cases of mysterious disease resembling Multiple Sclerosis. Until the early years of the 19th century, physicians relied on superstition and hearsay, to care for the ill. Medical ideas were never scientifically tested in the early 19th century. Physicians were often very good observers at that time and today we can look back and identify people who undoubtedly suffered from Multiple Sclerosis. These date back from writings as far back as the Middle Ages.

The first mention of this disease happened nearly 600 years earlier in the 1193 and was by Bishop Thorlak.  He described a young lady native from Iceland by the name Halldora, who lost her vision and movement suddenly. There were no explanation for this sudden event, and they resorted to prayers to the saints, and she miraculously recovered within seven days. She continued to have these mysterious symptoms for the next five years. With no further history on her, the cause of her death is still unknown.

There were no further writings in history about this disease for another two hundred years.

A Dutch nun, Saint Lidwina (1380–1433) of Schiedam, kept a journal of similar unexplained symptoms. This is the first documented case in history. From the age of 16 years old the nun was plagued by mysterious motor weakness, pain and vision loss until her death at the age of 53. This gave rise to the hypothesis that it is a "Viking Gene" responsible for the hardening of the nerve, as both were of Scandinavian descent.

Multiple Sclerosis is found frequently in Scandinavia, Iceland, the British Isles and the countries settled by their inhabitants and their descendants, i.e. the United States, Canada, Australia and New Zealand. This gave rise to the suggestion that the Vikings may have played an important role in spreading genetic susceptibility to the disease in these areas.  The Vikings raided most European countries, settling in Normandy, Southern Italy and Sicily, from where they traded with other parts of the world. These trade routes included parts of Northern Africa, the Black Sea, the Caspian Sea, India, and Persia and may have included China. They also migrated to the East and established the Russian state. The Varangians, a Viking related tribe became part of the Byzantine Empire. The Byzantine army was responsible for many a crusade in those years.  Together with the Mongolian Army, a regiment of Scandinavians they roamed through the entire European and Russian continent. Customary to their habit of capturing women and children and trading them as slaves gave increasing rise to this genetic dissemination in the early middle ages. Until this day, MS is known as a Viking disease.

The most famous case in history is that of Augustus Frederick d'Este (1794–1848), the grandson of King GoergeIII of England. In his well-documented diary he described all the typical symptoms of Multiple Sclerosis in a male.  The disease started its course with the onset of sudden vision loss, at the age of 28 while attending a funeral of a friend. His dairy spanned nearly 22 years, describing symptoms relating closely to Multiple Sclerosis. In his dairy he wrote about weakness of the legs, clumsiness of the hands, numbness, dizziness, bladder disturbances, and erectile dysfunction. But most noted is the mention of "Amaurosis fugax" or Latin for a sudden blindness in one eye over short periods of time. This is typically noted in Optic Neuritis in multiple Sclerosis. Augustus was wheelchair bound by the year of 1844, forty four years after his first episode.  He passed away 4 years later in 1848. Although his dairies stopped in 1846, he kept a positive outlook on life, and we can only deduce that he suffered very little cognitive dysfunction.

The British diarist W. N. P. Barbellion, a pen name of Bruce Frederick Cummings (1889–1919), maintained a dairy of his diagnosis and struggle with Multiple Sclerosis. His diary was published in 1919 under the title "The Journal of a Disappointed Man". He began his diaries as a young teenager, and by age 25 he had dedicated himself to their publication. The following year, in November 1915, Cummings was diagnosed with Multiple Sclerosis. The then unnamed disease played a significant role in his writing, and much of his published work contains reflections on his life with the debilitating illness. His most famous Quote: "the millions of bacteria gnawing away my precious spinal cord".

**Early historical medical findings of Multiple Sclerosis.**

Jean Cruveilhier (1791–1873), a French professor of pathologic anatomy, had detailed many of the disease's clinical aspects; however he never identified it as a separate disease. He was also the first to record the clinical history of a patient who had the disease. He published his findings in 1842, but never gave a name to this strange disease. He also did extensive studies on the inflammation of blood vessels, particularly phlebitis. He believed it to be the primary cause of diseases, and today phlebitis is a recognised symptom of Multiple Sclerosis.

Robert Carswell (1793–1857), a British professor of pathology and an artist also described Multiple Sclerosis before Charcot and drew detailed sketches of the plaques and lesion. He spent years in the hospitals and mortuaries of Paris and Lyon, painting watercolours and pen and ink drawings of patients and of post mortem preparations. Of the 1034 paintings, 99 are of the brain and spinal cords, and two are typical in the findings of Multiple Sclerosis. Carswell indicated he saw two examples of this pathology, although he never examined either patient, but illustrated one of them. The clinical histories of these patients were paralysis.

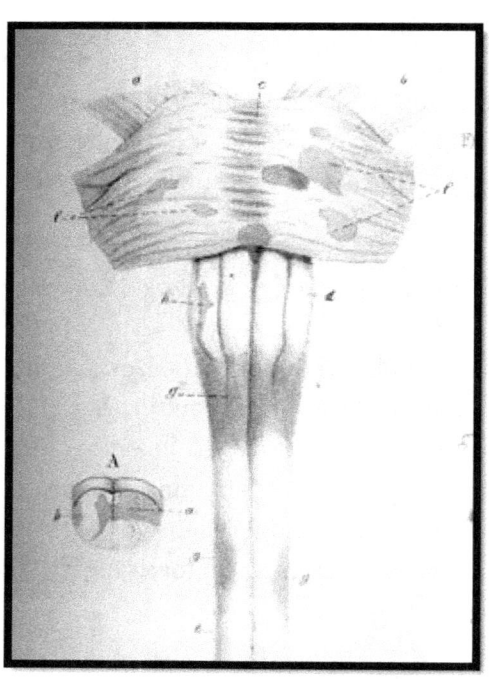

[9] Carswell drawings of Multiple Sclerosis Scarring.

The French neurologist Jean-Martin Charcot (1825–1893) was the first person to recognize multiple sclerosis as a distinct disease in 1868, calling this disease Sclerose en Plaque. The three signs of MS as described by him, now known as Charcot's triad 1 are nystagmus, intention tremor, and telegraphic speech (scanning speech). Charcot also observed cognition changes, describing his patients as having a "marked enfeeblement of the memory" and "conceptions that formed slowly". His first drawings from autopsies in 1983 and years to follow clearly indicated the scarring, typical of what is seen in modern medicine today. After Charcot's description, Eugène Devic (1858–1930), Jozsef Balo (1895–1979), Paul Ferdinand Schilder (1886–1940), and Otto Marburg (1874–1948) described different types of the disease. This is dealt with in the chapter for disease types in this book.

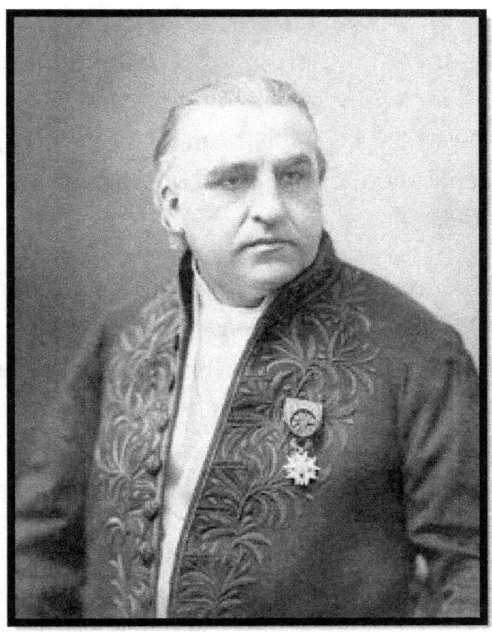

[10] Jean-Martin Charcot

Charcot, by then a professor at the University of Paris, has been was known as the father of modern Neurology. His first autopsy was done on a young woman whom he examined carefully while still living. He described tremors he had never seen before, and also noted other neurological problems including slurred speech and abnormal eye movement. Comparing this to other patients with similar symptoms, the decision was made to do an autopsy on her death. The autopsy showed signs of scarring to the brain tissues, describing them as Plaques. These scarring and plaques are similar to Multiple Sclerosis findings today.

As far as his treatment for this disease went, it led him to great frustration. This disease did not respond to any treatment even small doses of strychnine. Other treatments including the injection of tiny amounts of gold or silver, a treatment for nerve disorders in those years did not even help. The most common nerve disorder was Syphilis. The lack of symptomatic relieve by these treatments baffled Charcot.

In the 1880 one of the noted "physicians" was Doctor Sigmund Freud. His First Multiple Sclerosis patient was his former Nanny, who had Multiple Sclerosis. Freud in his infinite wisdom claimed "Creeping paralysis", as it was called in those days, was considered to be a mental condition caused by "female hysteria". This was a direct conclusion he drew from the fact that more females suffer from this disease than men. He firmly believed that he could cure MS by talking to his patient. Today it is this writer's opinion that some neurologists are still influenced by his thinking, hence the term Freudism in MS. His publication of Multiple Sclerosis is not consulted any more, and has been discredited over the years.

Louis-Antoine Ranvier (1835 –1922) was a French physician, pathologist, anatomist and histologist, who discovered nodes of Ranvier, regularly spaced discontinuities of the myelin sheath, occurring at varying intervals along the length of a nerve fibre. In 1867, Ranvier entered the Collège de France and worked as an assistant to Claude Bernard. In 1875, he was appointed to its chair of General Anatomy. In 1878, he discovered the nodes of Ranvier or Myelin as it is now known as. This finding is of particular significance as the sheath that protects our nerve axons consist of myelin.

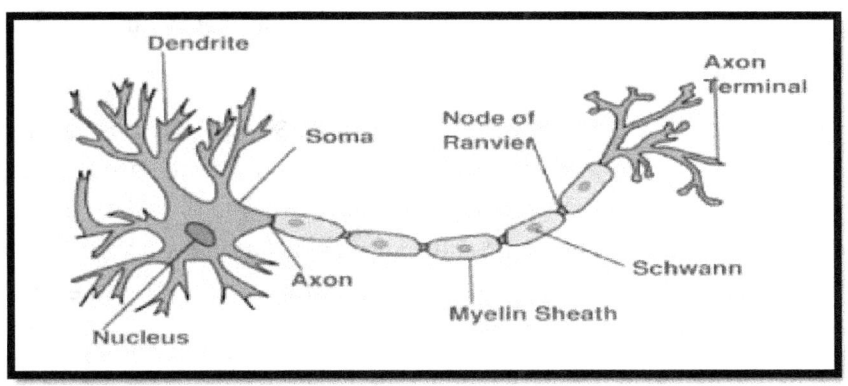

[11] Nodes of Ranvier (Image source: National Library of Medicine (NLM))

Dr Louis Ranvier discovered the nodes which received his name. Other anatomical structures bearing his name are the Merkel-Ranvier cells, melanocyte-like cells in the basal layer of the epidermis that contain catecholamine granules; and Ranvier's tactile disks, a special type of sensory nerve ending. Node of Ranvier is a periodic gap in the insulating sheath (myelin) on the axon of certain neurons that serves to facilitate the rapid conduction of nerve impulses. The Myelin sheath acts as a high-resistance, low-capacitance electrical insulator. However, nodes of Ranvier interrupt the insulation at intervals, and this discontinuity enables impulses to jump from node to node in a process known as salutatory conduction.

Georg Eduard von Rindfleisch (1836 – 1908) was a German pathologist. Rindfleisch was the first to note that inflammation may play a role in Multiple Sclerosis. His first writings were in 1863, where he noted the inflammation spreads through the central nervous system from veins spreading outwards. In other words, the demyelination process starts from the veins outwards. This was the first notion that Multiple Sclerosis may be an inflammatory disease, although the source of the inflammation was never mentioned. His work was the background for the later Tracy Putnam work's on the vascular theory of Multiple Sclerosis. Five years later Charcot named the disease Sclerose en Plaques.

In the last decades of the 19th century, most leading physicians came to understand that MS was a specific disease in the world. MS was recognized in England by Dr Walter Moxon in 1873 and in the United States by Dr Edward Seguin in 1878. By the late 19th century, much of what can be learned about MS clinical characteristics was known. The disease is more common in women than men, that it is not directly inherited and that it can produce many different neurological symptoms.

By the late 19th century little was known about Multiple Sclerosis and as to what was the cause of it and for the lack of better diagnostic equipment, research was basically at a standstill. The notion of it being an auto immune disorder was not even considered, as the very existence of auto immune disease was not known in those years. Multiple Sclerosis was by then suspected as a result of the body withholding sweat, and was treated with herbs.

Bacteria were first noted as a cause for diseases by the late 19th century. In the early 20th century even smaller organisms, viruses became known to physicians. Techniques were developed to study these viruses and bacteria by growing them in laboratories. In 1906 Dr Camillo Golgi and Dr Santiago Ramon Y Cajal were awarded the Nobel Prize for medicine for the perfection of chemicals to enhance the visibility of cells under the microscope.

Dr James Dawson at the University of Edinburgh used this technology to perform a detailed microscopic examination of patient who died due to MS. In 1916 he described the Dawson fingers in Multiple Sclerosis and this was later confirmed by Charles Lumsden and credits his work to Dawson findings. Dawson described the spread of Finger like lesions or plaques from the ventricles outwards. He also noted the spread of inflammation from the veins in the ventricles outwards.

In the ten years after the World War 1 with research growing more sophisticated the first abnormalities was found in the spinal fluid of Multiple Sclerosis patients. This was first noted in 1919. Myelin, described by DR. Ranvier in 1878, was studied under the microscope and this led to the discovery of the cells that make up the myelin in 1928. Oligodendrocytes principle function is to provide support to axons and to produce the Myelin sheath. In 1943, the actual composition of myelin was determined.

Lord Edgar Douglas Adrian (1889 –1977) established a technique to measure electrical nerve impulses in 1925. This device Electroencephalograph (EEG) records of electrical activity along the scalp. EEG measures voltage fluctuations resulting from ionic current flows within the neurons of the brain. In clinical contexts, EEG refers to the recording of the brain's spontaneous electrical activity over a short period of time. The resulting knowledge included clarification of the role of myelin in nerve conduction and a realization that demyelinated nerves cannot transmit impulses efficiently. A Nobel Prize of peace was awarded to him in 1932 for this ground breaking work. Today this technique is used widely in different forms in the diagnoses of Multiple Sclerosis.

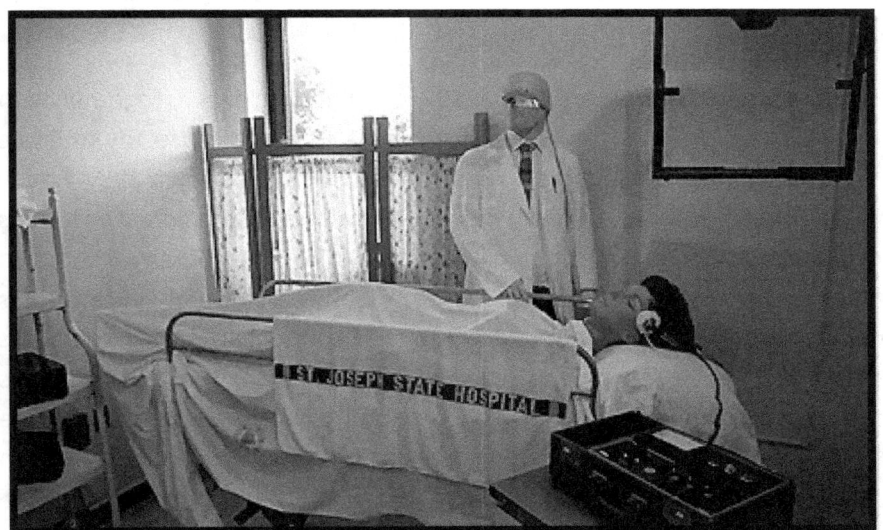

[12] Electroencephalograph

During this time, scientists suspected that Multiple Sclerosis was caused by some form of toxin or poison. Due to the fact that MS damage occurs around the blood vessels it was believed that toxins circulating in the blood stream leaked out into the brain, but no researcher was able to pinpoint this.

Just before the outbreak of the Second World War research on vaccines provided an important breakthrough for MS researchers. Persons vaccinated for viral disease, especially rabies, sometime lead to a disease that closely resembled Multiple Sclerosis. It was assumed that because the vaccine was not completely inactive, it attacked Myelin.

Dr Thomas Milton Rivers (1888 –1962) an American bacteriologist and virologist at the Rockefeller Institute in New York City, demonstrated that immune cells and not viruses were the cause of Multiple Sclerosis. This led to the birth of the animal model of multiple sclerosis in 1935. Using virus free laboratory animals, he injected myelin into them. This led to the laboratory specimens to develop MS like symptoms with the immune symptom attacking the animals Myelin. This animal form of MS, called experimental allergic encephalomyelitis, or EAE, became the base for the animal model being used and still used today. The animal model was largely over looked in those years as it was still presumed that toxins were the cause and these were still studied. Dr Rivers became known as the father of modern virology.

In the 1930's Tracy Jackson Putnam (1894–1975) multiple sclerosis, together with Alexandra Adler were the first people to propose a vascular cause for multiple sclerosis, resurrecting the previous works of Eduard von Rindfleisch. In 1937 Tracey Putman and Alexandra Adler specifically described that cerebral plaques or lesions developed closely to the large epiventrical veins in the brain. They also demonstrated distortions on the veins near the lesion area. Putman indicated this link to Multiple Sclerosis in the 1930's, and even tried to replicate this in dogs. This replication was done by injecting obstructing agents in the longitudinal sinus veins of dogs. The obstructing agents consisted of lard oil. The lesions that were demonstrated after this experiment were similar to Multiple Sclerosis, although not exactly, being that they resembled more the damage caused by a mini stroke than Multiple Sclerosis. The assumption followed that Multiple Sclerosis was a vascular disease and patients were treated by blood thinners or anticoagulants.

Probably the biggest influence in Multiple Sclerosis was the introduction of the National Multiple Sclerosis Society in 1946. It was founded by Sylvia Lawry (1915–2001), whose brother suffered from the disease. After placing an advertisement in the New York Times, enquiring if anyone else has recovered from this disease. The feedback she received was not what she was expected. Instead she got flooded by letters from patient who suffered from MS. Instead of being discouraged, she mobilized a group of friends and advisors, including some who had answered her ad. This was the start of the National MS Society. Their aim was to promote contacts among neurologists around the country who treated MS and to raise money to fund a search for answers.

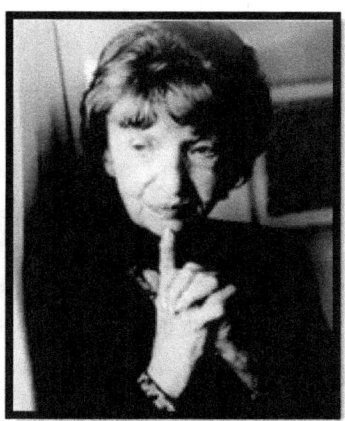

[13] Sylvia Lawry

The famous add consisted of 11 words. "Multiple Sclerosis. Will anyone recovered from it please communicate with patient," Sylvia Lawry stated in the New York Times. This was Sylvia Lawry's first step in the fight for a world without Multiple Sclerosis. Famous scientists joined her cause and by 1946 the US National MS society was formed followed in 1967 by the worldwide Multiple Sclerosis International Federation (MSIF) in London. The MSIF coordinates a network of national MS societies and the international MS research community. The MSIF is a driving force behind worldwide research not only to find effective and financially feasible therapies but also a cure for the disease. In 2001 the Federation founded the Sylvia Lawry Centre for Multiple Sclerosis Research in Munich. The MSIF supports the creation and further development of new and existing MS societies.

The first research grant from the then called "The Society for the Advancement of Multiple Sclerosis Research", was awarded funding for the study of immunology of Multiple Sclerosis. This grant was awarded to study the relationship between the body's immune system and the central nervous system.

Dr Elvin Kabat at Columbia University who discovered abnormalities in the spinal fluid in MS patients received this grant in 1947.This consisted of abnormal immunologic proteins in the spinal fluid and appeared in patterns known as Oligoclonal bands. The presence of Oligoclonal bands in the spinal fluid is a major indication of MS and also demonstrates that the immune system and MS is connected.

Through the work of the National MS Society research in multiple sclerosis expanded rapidly over the decades that followed.

In 1953, a major medical breakthroughs of the century occurred with the Nobel Prize-winning description of DNA by Dr Francis Crick and Dr James Watson. This led to the understanding of how genes control biologic functions; including the role genetics played in the immune system. In 1960 the NMSS had also adopted and introduced the Schumacher Criteria for diagnosis of Multiple Sclerosis. This resulted in the creation of a panel of experts, appointed by the NMMS, under the guidance of Dr Schumacher. At the same time, a rating scale to determine the level of disability caused by MS was developed by Dr John Kurtzke.

In 1960 the doctors believed that Multiple Sclerosis was caused by some sort of allergic reaction and the patients were treated with vitamins and antihistamines. During the 1950 -60s, the first major breakthrough was discovered in Multiple Sclerosis and with the ability to make more accurate diagnosis it was possible to begin proper scientific test on MS. The first successful trial was the use of adrenocorticotropic hormone (ACTH) in treating this disease. A group of patients that were in active relapse were given ACTH while a control group, also in relapse, was given a placebo  or in plain English a substance with no medicinal value. In 1969 the results of this trial proved that patients treated with ACTH recovered far quicker than those on the placebo. ACTH which is a hormone normally produced by the pituitary gland stimulates the adrenal glands to produce more natural steroids. The outcome was that this overproduction of natural steroids provides an anti-inflammatory effect, while supressing the immune system. ACTH was later replaced by high dose IV steroids and is still today the mainline treatment for a relapse.

In the 1960s, scientific research into the cause of MS focused on two main theories that are still being explored today. The immune system was studied intensively and the white blood cells that attack myelin were investigated. Myelin basic protein, were discovered in both EAE and human MS, and the indication was that the immune system attacks this protein. The possibility that MS involves a direct immune-system attack on myelin was investigated.

The next idea stemmed from studies that showed that people with MS have altered antibodies against viruses. The old belief that MS could be caused by a virus was also revisited. Rather than thinking a viral infection was directly damaging the central nervous system, it was rather considered that viruses involved in MS altered the immune system and this triggers the attacks that damages myelin.

Today, it is still considered that MS is a combination of infectious and an autoimmune disease. All of the treatments that were developed for MS target either an infectious or an immune reaction.

The first Computed Axial Tomography (CAT) scans were performed in 1978 on Multiple Sclerosis patients. The Nobel Prize was awarded to Allan McLeod Cormack and Sir Godfrey Hounsfield in 1979. Hounsfield invented the first commercially viable CT scanner in 1967.

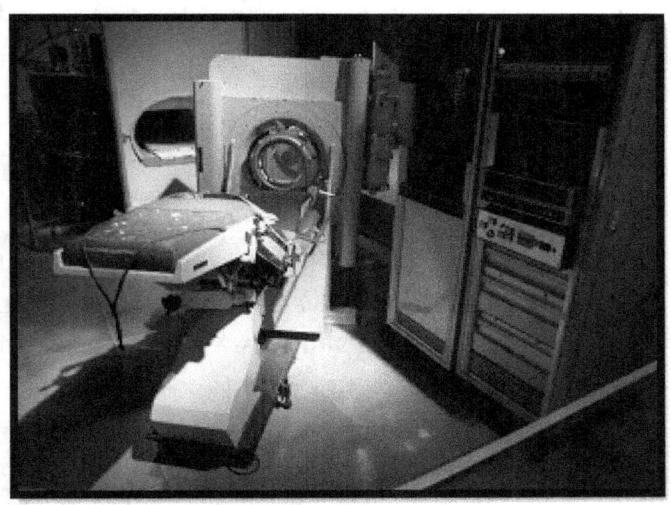

[14] Historical EMI Scanner. (Image source: Wikipedia. Author: Philipcosson)

The first EMI-Scanner was installed in Atkinson Morley Hospital in Wimbledon, England, and the first patient brain-scan was done on 1 October 1971. The first EMI scanner, as it was first known was installed in the USA at the Mayo Clinic, a clinic now famous for research on Multiple Sclerosis. The original 1971 prototype took 160 parallel readings through 180 angles, each 1° apart, with each scan taking a little over 5 minutes. The images from these scans took 2.5 hours to be processed by algebraic reconstruction techniques on a large computer. Today the computer and the scanner itself are more involved and scanning and computing times are largely reduced.

This decade was also the first time Evoke Potential tests were used to measure nerve conduction in Multiple Sclerosis. This test is a result of the advancement in the electroencephalography (EEG) and electromyography (EMG) tests. In 1965, Spehlmann used a checkerboard stimulation to describe human Visual Evoke Potential tests (VEPs). The first attempt to localize structures in the visual pathway was completed by Szikla and his colleagues. Halliday and colleagues completed the first investigations using VEP by recording delayed VEPs in a patient with optic neuritis in 1972. Shortly after that followed Sensory Evoke Potential test (SEP) and Brainstem Auditory Evoked Potential test (BAEP). This is widely used in diagnosing MS and its symptoms today.

In 1970 while studying EAE or the animal model of Multiple Sclerosis, it was suspected that some myelin proteins released by cells prevented the disease and actually seemed to protect the animals. The first product was named copolymer1 and is today an approved disease-modifying drug named Copaxone.

By the late 1970, we also saw the first studies on interferons now widely used in reducing MS attacks or Flare ups.

During the 1980- 1990s, new treatment trials began in earnest and more detail became available as to how white blood cells are activated to start an immune attack on myelin. Researchers also noted that some viruses are similar to human tissue and an immune response can cause the body to attack its own cells, seeing them as foreign invaders. A virus can also set off such an attack or immune response with the body attacking its own cells while fighting a viral infection. This also led scientist to believe that Multiple Sclerosis may be caused by a disease and one of these may be the Epstein Bar Virus.

The white blood cell type that actually causes the damage in Multiple Sclerosis was also identified. Although Macrophages were discovered by Ilya Mechnikov, a Russian bacteriologist, in 1884 it was the first time Macrophages were noted as the culprit. Macrophages are derived from the Greek word meaning the "big eater" and are cells produced by the changing of monocytes (white blood cells) into tissues. When a monocyte enters damaged tissue through the endothelium of a blood vessel, it undergoes a series of changes to become a macrophage. In

Multiple Sclerosis, the Blood Brain Barrier is supposed to stop monocytes from crossing into the brain.

In this decade we also saw the first study of Multiple Sclerosis in twins and the role that genetics plays in MS. The twin of a person with MS very rarely develops MS as well, indicating that genes have only a partial role to play in MS. However that being said, we know that genetics plays a role as MS is found to be more common in persons with MS in their ancestor or direct family.

These were the years that saw the introduction of the MRI scanner. Magnetic resonance imaging (MRI) is a major diagnostic tool used to image the body's soft tissue, and in the case of Multiple Sclerosis, it is used to create remarkable clarity of the brain and spinal cord. Dr Raymond Damadian, an Armenian-American physician, scientist, and professor at the Downstate Medical Center State University of New York, created the world's first magnetic resonance imaging machine in 1972.

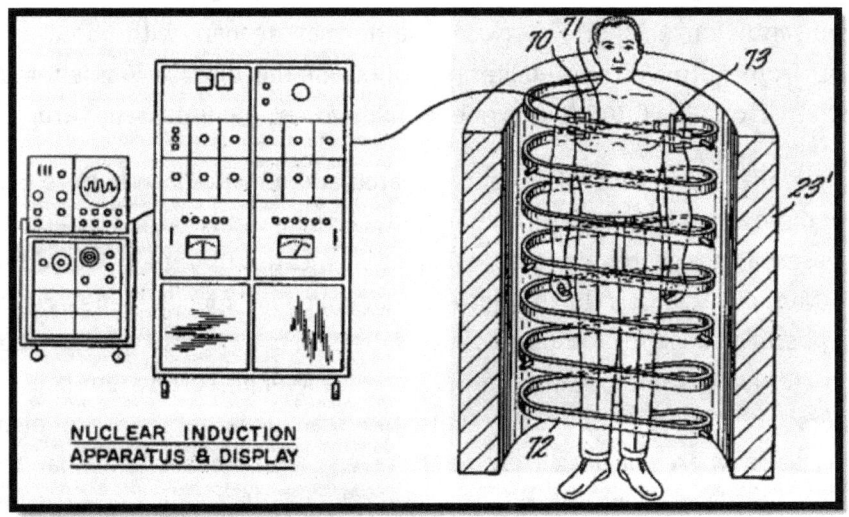

[15] Prototype for the first MRI scanner.

A medical breakthrough was made with the first MRI scan that was done in 1981 by DR I R Young in England. By 1984 the MRI scanner was able to detect a Multiple Sclerosis attack in the brain and was also able to detect MS attacks in the brain without the patient actually showing signs of a relapse. By 1988 significant advances in MRI technology changed the way MS was perceived. It was now noted that MS is a constant on-going disease even though the patient shows no signs of a relapse.

During the 1980 till today, major trails were begun on many drugs to treat Multiple Sclerosis and the first drug was commercially released that effectively slowed down MS disease progression. This would not have been possible without the guidance and assistance of the National Multiple Sclerosis Society.

The nineties was the era of the brain and clinical break-through and more sophisticated diagnostic equipment created a much clearer picture of Multiple Sclerosis. Enter the computer era as well and database and information was shared over a broader spectrum. The MRI Scanner has rapidly reduced the actual diagnosis time from 7 years in 1970 to 6 months currently.

The initial research on drugs started bearing fruit and the majority of MS symptoms could now be treated, and we also saw the introduction of the disease modifying drugs including Interferons. The average life span of a Multiple Sclerosis patient was now significantly longer and fairly close to a normal lifespan, with about a 5 year reduction from normal. The debilitating course of the disease was altered drastically with the so called CRAB (Copaxone, Rebif, Avonex and Betaseron) drugs.

The nineties was also the decade of genetic research and an American led project to decode and discover all genes in the human body, also focused on the role genes played in diseases. The research done on twins also indicated that genes played a major role in Multiple Sclerosis. In the decade that followed specific genes were targeted as a possible cause for Multiple Sclerosis. Scientists have also now shifted their focus on stem cell treatment or in other genetically engineered stem cell to alter the course of Multiple Sclerosis. Plasmapheresis treatments were also introduced in cases where all drug treatments failed. This process is similar to kidney dialysis with blood being filtered and the Killer t-cells being removed by special filters.

Today we are on the eve of major advances in curing and halting this debilitating disease in its tracks. During the period 1993 to 2004 we saw the release of 6 new drugs to modify the disease path and increase our ability to move and function. Before this there were no disease modifying drugs on the market. An old favourite, that Multiple Sclerosis is a vascular disease is also now again in the spotlight, and only time will tell if it will bear fruit or not. The first so called vaccine is in trail phase and the next couple of years we might be able to halt this disease or even cure it.

Rapid advancement is being made to effectively treat this disease, and we owe a huge debt of gratitude to Sylvia Lawry with the creation of the body of the National Multiple Sclerosis Society. Without this body and dedicated scientists and doctors over the world we would have been far from a possible cure.

# What is Multiple Sclerosis?

Multiple Sclerosis is a disease and is not contagious.  This I have read in many literature, and been told by many neurologists. Most likely MS occurs as a result of some combination of genetic, environmental and infectious factors, and possibly other factors like vascular problems. It is not considered a hereditary disease but the risk of acquiring MS is higher in relatives of a person with the disease than in the general populations. Epidemiological studies of MS have provided hints on possible causes for the disease. Theories try to combine the known data into plausible explanations, but none has proved definitive. It is what is called an auto-immune disease, although this is not confirmed as it is still considered suspected. . There are theories that it may be caused by a virus, and I will get into these later. But for now let's dwell on the theory that it is an auto-immune disease.

The name Auto immune Diseases arises from the body's natural immune response attacking its own cells, seeing these cells as foreign invaders. There are a couple of factors that starts this unhealthy immune response, and top of the list is a simple reaction to an immune response to common cold or flu. The body's immune response will first attack the flu or cold, but will then move into overdrive mode and attack healthy cells in the body. In Multiple Sclerosis (MS) this unhealthy immune response sees the myelin sheath, the sheath that protects the neural pathways in the brain and spinal cord, as a foreign invader and it attacks the myelin on the long axons of the nerve.

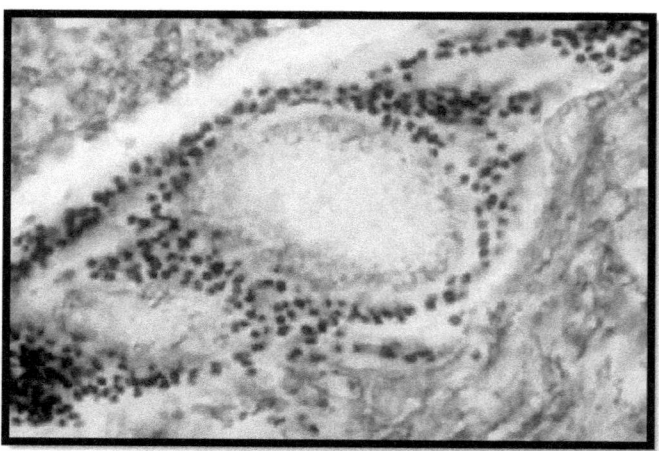

[16] Myelin Damage in (Image Source: CDC/Dr. Karp, Emory University)

Myelin consists of about 40% water, with a dry mass of lipids or fat cells, and protein make up to 30 – 40% of Myelin. The purpose of myelin is to insulate the nerve axons from losing electrical impulses, the energy source that drives the brain function. For each command the brain issues or receives, an electrical impulse or impulses are sent to the muscle nerve controls to act in a certain manner or carry out a certain function and vice versa. Impulses are also sent back to the brain in a similar function. The whole human body is controlled by electrical impulses. The more protection there is along the sheath of the nerve axons the better off we are.

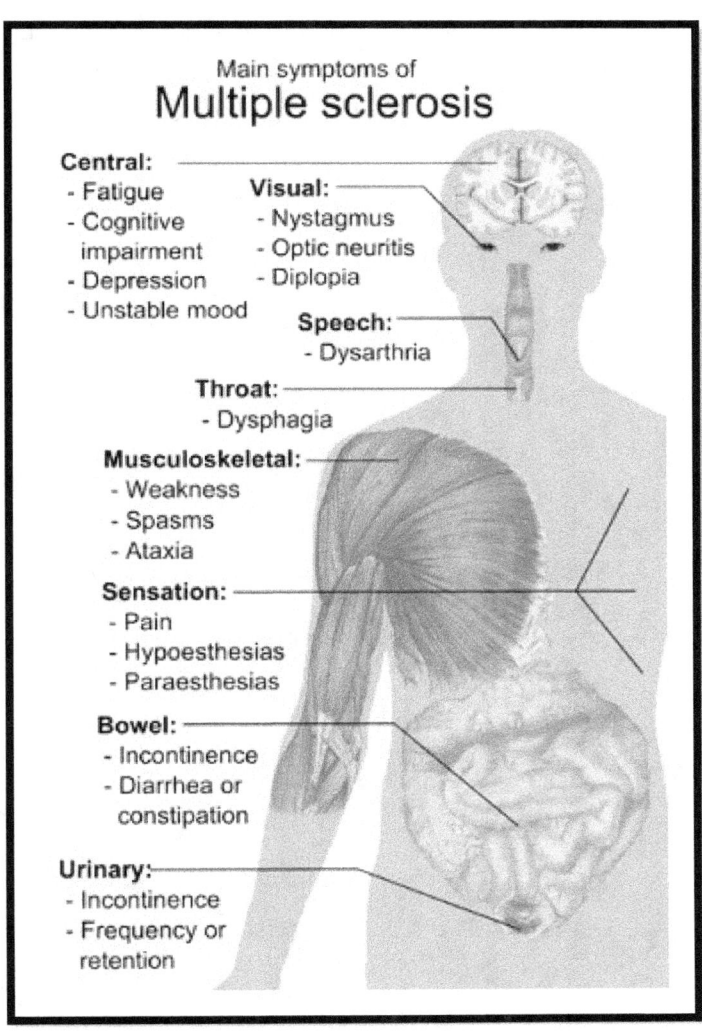

[17] Multiple Sclerosis Symptoms (Image source: Wikipedia. Author: Mikael Häggström)

However when we remove this protection, we lose transmission of this electrical impulses, either by the impulses just leaving the nerve axon and not reaching the intended end point, or by it shorting from one axon to another terminating the impulse at that point. A good example would be either a damage electrical cable in your home losing its ability to transmit electricity or a short between two wires because the insulation is stripped. Myelin is our electrical insulation cover over our electrical wire system, the nerve axon.  The body's immune system is attacking this myelin sheath and seeing it as an enemy in your body. The attack causes the myelin sheath to be stripped of the protective sheave, and causing an electrical impulse malfunction due to the damage done by the immune system malfunction.

# The different types of Multiple Sclerosis

There are four main types of Multiple Sclerosis and in 1996 the National Multiple Sclerosis Society standardized four clinical courses. There are also three subtypes of Multiple Sclerosis. Clinically isolated Syndrome or CIS is one episode of a relapse and the symptoms never appear again.

Relapsing Remitting Multiple sclerosis or RRMS is normally the first stage of multiple sclerosis where the patient suffers from intermittent relapses or flare ups. During a relapse the symptoms of multiple sclerosis appear. The symptoms can be either new symptoms or old symptoms that re-appear. Normally after a relapse the symptoms disappear totally, or the patient may retain a little of the symptom. After each relapse, the remission stage will follow. RRMS accounts for about 85% of Multiple Sclerosis patients.

During the remission stage these symptoms disappear completely within a matter of time. The extent of time for these symptoms to subside differs from person to person. Where there are old symptoms that remain during the remission stage they tend to worsen with the next relapse. In the early stages of Multiple Sclerosis the symptoms normally disappears for days, weeks, months or years before they reappear. Each relapse will follow with a remission stage where the patient is nearly symptom free. This type of Multiple Sclerosis is referred to as RRMS or relapse remitting Multiple Sclerosis. It presents itself in early adult hood in most cases, but may appear later in life, even at an age of 40 years or older.

One of the classic hallmarks of RRMS is the variability of its symptoms and no two are affected by the same set of symptoms in the same way. Symptoms appears only to disappear again with or without treatment, however corticosteroids is used in most cases to treat the relapse. The symptoms of RRMS and any other form of MS are quite wide spread, and include the following.

- Numbness and tingling

- Radiating pain, like a mild electrical shock, when bending the neck

- Sensitivity to heat

- Dizziness

- Bowel or bladder problems

- Eye pain and vision problems such as double vision or jerky vision, and this today is recognised as the first symptom of Multiple Sclerosis

- Sexual Dysfunction

- Difficulty walking moving and  muscle stiffness

- General weakness and fatigue

- Problems with balance and coordination

- Depression or mood swings

- Cognitive dysfunction effecting thoughts and expressions.

A typical RRMS relapse or "Flare up" can last anywhere from 24 hours to several weeks. An attack can involves one or many of the symptoms. A flare up may worsen existing problems or cause the development of new symptoms. Remission between flare ups in some cases can last for years. My first period of remission lasted nearly 4 years in the beginning. An important factor to remember is to keep a close eye on symptoms, and inform your Doctor as soon as possible. Do not wait for it for symptoms to disappear on its own, as the lasting effect of a flare up can be very devastating. The old saying applies here, "Prevention is far better than cure". Rather get treatment, be it a horrible experience for some, than to lose an important function to operate a day to day life.

Secondary Progressive Multiple Sclerosis normally follows RRMS.  With Secondary Progressive Multiple Sclerosis or SPMS, the symptoms that are present, steadily worsen over a period of time with each new attack or flare up. With SPMS there are no or few remitting stages and the patient steadily worsens over time. The symptoms are here to stay and very few medications do slow down the progression of the disease.

With SPMS the patient will have good days and bad days, with a variety of external factors playing a role in the disease. Examples are heat and diet and other factors like stress and over activity play a role in how the patient may feel. These factors may worsen the symptoms. In this type of Multiple Sclerosis, the patient will suffer more and more relapses, with nearly no remission that follows the relapses. This type of MS normally appears after a 10-15 years of Multiple Sclerosis, but it is not to say that all RRMS patient will develop Secondary Progressive Multiple Sclerosis. SPMS develops in about 65% of all Multiple Sclerosis patients. The disease will progress more steadily, but not necessary more rapidly.

When the so called "CRAB" drugs (Copaxone, Rebif, Avonex and Betaseron) or other disease modifying drugs do not tend to slow down the progression in Multiple Sclerosis, it is evident that the patient is moving from RRMS to SPMS. Upon treating a relapse with corticosteroids, and the result being only a small decrease in symptoms or none at all is a definite indicator of SPMS. A change in relapse timing and degree of severity increasing, and the ability to recover from such relapses is a clear sign of moving from RRMS to SPMS. In SPMS the relapses will tend to disappear, and the disease will run a devastating course with more progression without relapse. In other words the brain axons or nerve endings are losing its ability to repair and are destroyed on a continual basis.

The Expanded Disability Status Scale (EDDS), a scale used to measure the severity of MS, comes into play here as well. RRMS tend to have a score of four or less while patients with SPMS normally have a score of six or higher. Patients with RRMS upon reaching 4 to 5.5 tend to develop SPMS in a very short period of time. An EDDS in that range means the patent has difficulty walking 500m meters. And require some assisted devices or a cane, and a rest period as severe fatigue sets in. The EDDS scale will be discussed in detail later. SPMS patients also have higher incidents of cognitive disability or higher brain functions impairment. Also present is the appearance of more lesions or plaques on the brain. However, there is normally a decrease in gadolinium-enhancing lesions (contrast enhancing), due to the absence of less inflammation of the brain.  There is more degenerative damage in the form of damage to the nerve endings developing more unhealed scarring.

Progressive Relapsing Multiple Sclerosis is as the title describes, progressive relapsing multiple sclerosis or PRMS. The relapses are more frequent and there is less remission between each relapse. During each relapse, the symptoms steadily worsen with new symptoms appearing with new attacks sometimes. There is normally no recovery from the symptoms and they are permanent. This is the debilitating stage of multiple sclerosis. This phase normally appears also about 10-15 years after the initial onset of MS. PRMS is not basically used often to classify this type of MS any more, but rather PPMS or SPMS, depending on the frequency of the attacks.

Primary Progressive Multiple Sclerosis is the basic type of MS and most MS sufferers are in this stage. The onset leads to continuous worsening of each attack. Unfortunately there is no remission periods in this type, and with each attack there is a continual worsening of the symptoms. The severity of the symptoms may differ from each attack but there are always lasting effects from the attacks.

This type is the most common and is only diagnosed in the age group of 30 - 50. More men than women are diagnosed with this type of MS first.

Progressive Relapsing Multiple Sclerosis (PRMS) is as the title describes, progressive relapsing Multiple Sclerosis or PRMS. Progressive relapsing MS describes those individuals who, from onset, have a steady neurologic decline but also suffer more severe attacks. This is the least common of all subtypes. The relapses are more frequent and there is less remission between each relapse. During each relapse the symptoms steadily worsen with new symptoms appearing with new attacks occasionally. There is normally a certain extent of recovery from the symptoms but the after effects of the relapse are there to stay, with little or no recovery. This is a debilitating stage of Multiple Sclerosis. PRMS is not basically used often to classify this type of MS anymore; however emphasis is placed on this form of MS, but rather PPMS or SPMS, depending on the frequency of the attack. PRMS is prevalent in about 5% of all MS patients.

Primary Progressive Multiple Sclerosis (PPMS) is the distinct from normal Multiple Sclerosis. The onset leads to continuous worsening and is characterized by no relapses, exacerbations or attacks. Unfortunately there are no remissions from this type and there is a continual worsening of the neurologic functions. The severity of the symptoms may differ in patients, from mild to very severe worsening. More men than women are diagnosed with this type of MS first. This type is the most common and is only diagnosed in the age group of 30 - 50. The absence of relapses or attacks makes PPMS less predictable than normal MS. The prevalence of this type of MS is about 15% of all MS patients.

Patients with primary progressive MS experience this very differently than normal MS Patients. Unlike people with other forms of MS, who have attacks followed by symptom-free periods, there are no relapses or attacks, but only a gradual worsening of symptoms. Being diagnosed with this type of MS does not paint a rosy picture, but rather a grim outlook. Certain studies indicate that most PPMS patient will need aid in walking after 7 years, and may be much debilitated after 10-15 years. The period from diagnosis to being completely bedridden is about 25 years which is reality in 75% of PPMS patients.

There's no "bright side" to primary progressive MS. But the absence of sudden attacks may make primary progressive MS slightly less unpredictable than other forms of MS, which can strike suddenly and severely. The most common symptoms are leg weakness, leg stiffness and difficulty walking and the spinal cord involvement is slightly higher in PPMS patient. A history of visual problems in the early stages of life has been noted in some cases.

Understanding what type of Multiple Sclerosis you have will help a lot in the treatment of your disease. The above classification is used to correctly treat your MS and helps you manage the disease.

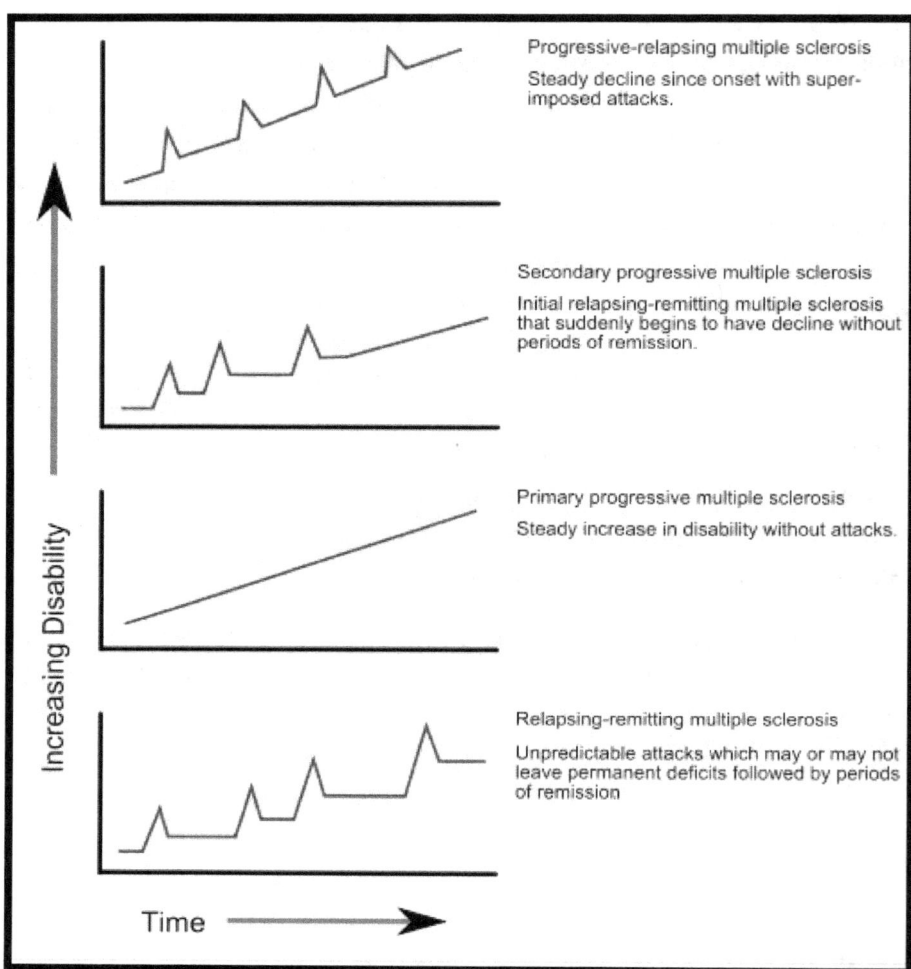

[18] Progression of Multiple Sclerosis Type (Image source: Wikipedia. Author: GetThePapersGetThePapers)

Apart from the four above types of Multiple Sclerosis there are other sub types of Multiple Sclerosis as well.

**The subtypes of Multiple Sclerosis**

Benign Multiple Sclerosis is a subtype of Multiple Sclerosis. Benign Multiple Sclerosis normally only affects the sensory system and in certain cases it could also affect the motor function of the patient. It follows the normal pattern of Multiple Sclerosis in the beginning, but after the first attack you are completely back to normal. There may be some relapses but it is spaced far apart, sometimes up to 10-15 years. The classification on the expanded disability status scale is less than two. Some patients may never have a flare-up or attack again and remain symptom free for the rest of their life. The prevalence of this type is very low with on average, only 5% being diagnosed with this type of Multiple Sclerosis. Benign MS patients, contrary to typical MS patients, hardly develop any physical disabilities at all.

Most neurologists don't use this term, but rather refer to it as mild multiple sclerosis. The risk is still there to develop normal multiple sclerosis in life, and in some cases these patients do develop multiple sclerosis later in life. Disease modifying drugs are hardly ever given to these types of MS patients, sparing them the side effects of the so called "CRAB" drugs, but it always a big question as to when to give disease modifying drugs. A good neurologist will only give disease modifying drugs after the first two relapses, depending as to how far apart they are spaced, after ruling out the possibility of Benign Multiple Sclerosis.

In Europe on a project called "MAGNIMS"', a collaboration of Magnetic Resonance Imaging (MRI) imaging experts are partaking in a study comparing a large amount of MRI data. MAGNIMS researchers have found certain cognitive impairment in Benign MS patients. This figure is as high as 45% in early studies, and the conclusion is to first rule this out before diagnosing a Benign Multiple Sclerosis.

There is also one very big drawback to this type of MS, and again I am stepping on some toes here. The biggest advocacy group of alternative treatments consist of this type of patients. MS is a disease that drives fear into people, and we all hope for some form or the other treatment to rid us of this monster, and a tendency exists to believe any so-called treatment, being it complete bogus or not. In the forefront of this are patients claiming they have been cured by this or that treatment, with little or none scientific data to back up this data. The majority of this group do actually consist of benign patients, secondary to patients having long time periods between relapses. Rather trust your neurologist on treatment than this group of people, primarily found on the internet.

**Diffuse myelinoclastic sclerosis** or "Schilder's Disease" (named after Paul F. Schilder who first describes it in 1912) is a tumour like sclerosis that forms one or two large demyelinating lesions on the brain. These lesion are normally larger than normal Multiple Sclerosis. It is a very infrequent disease, but because it is similar to multiple sclerosis, it is referred to as borderline Multiple Sclerosis. This type of Multiple Sclerosis normally only appears in children from the age of 4 - 15 years old, but it can sometimes appear in adults as well. Currently the youngest child ever to be diagnosed is 8 months old.

The symptom of this is similar to normal Multiple Sclerosis but also include dementia, seizures, trouble swallowing, personality changes and poor attention span. Other symptoms are similar to normal Multiple Sclerosis.

Like multiple sclerosis it has three types. It may be once off attack and never relapse again, relapse remitting or progressive with increase disability problems. The treatment of this in children consists basically of steroids as the disease modifying drugs are not tested for use in children yet. In adults, the treatment is the same as normal multiple sclerosis. Children who do suffer from this type normally don't have a good prognosis and are normally very disabled by the time they reach the age of twenty.

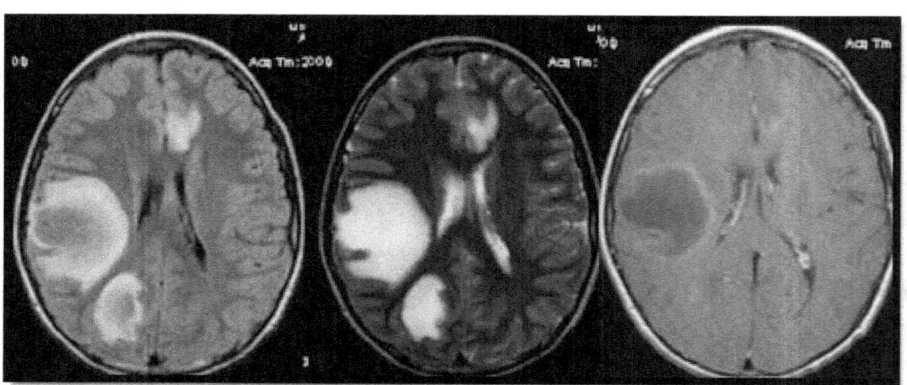

[19] Typical Schilder's Disease MRI Image (Image source: National Library of Medicine (NLM))

The Poser criteria* for diagnosing Diffuse Myelinoclastic Sclerosis or "Schilder's Disease" are as follows.

- One or two roughly symmetrical large plaques. Plaques are greater than 2 cm diameter.

- No other lesions are present and there are no abnormalities of the peripheral nervous system.

- Results of adrenal function studies and serum very long chain fatty acids are normal.

- Pathological analysis is consistent with sub-acute or chronic myelinoclastic diffuse sclerosis.

* P.S. Be patient on the Poser Criteria, I will get to it later in this chapter.

**Malignant Multiple Sclerosis** is a very aggressive form of Multiple Sclerosis. They call it Marburg's variant named after Otto Marburg (1874 – 1948) an Austrian neurologist. Marburg is a fulminant form of MS characterized by severe inflammation in the brain. In less technical terms it means occurring suddenly and with great intensity or severity.  The onset of this type of multiple sclerosis is normally preceded by a fever and mostly effects younger patients. It is a very rare form of multiple sclerosis that attacks the long axon of the nerves. Marburg's variant is also known as acute multiple sclerosis. The onset is very rapid with no remission. It was considered a fatal type of Multiple Sclerosis but it can be controlled in some cases with Alemtuzumab, Cyclophosphamide and Mitoxantrone. High dose corticosteroids are used frequently used in this type of Multiple Sclerosis.

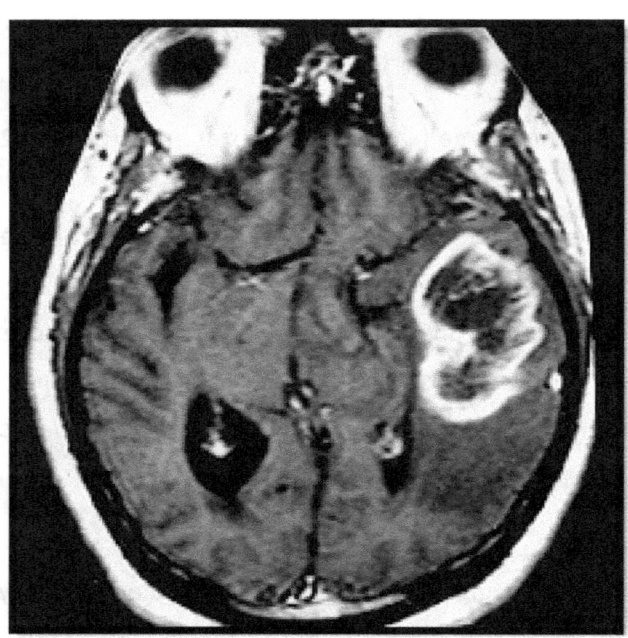

[20] Typical Marburg's lesion. Image source: (Wikipedia. Credit: The Armed Forces Institute of Pathology)

Marburg's Multiple Sclerosis is associated with a very large area of the cerebrum or big brain being affected by rather large lesions. Marburg is a lethal form of Multiple Sclerosis with the normal life expectancy being about five years, but with modern medicine the lifespan can be extended rather significantly. Due to the aggressiveness of this form of MS, debilitating symptoms are very high, with patients ending up with very severe disabilities in a very short time span.

Marburg's variant of Multiple Sclerosis is also called Tumefactive Multiple Sclerosis due to the large size of the lesions in the brain. As can be seen from the picture above, the scaring is very large and in a contrast enhanced MRI it is clearly visible as a large area of inflammation in the brain. The term Tumefactive is coined from its similar image make up of a tumour in the brain. The lesion size can vary from about 2cm to very large areas with a mass effect causing pressure on the surrounding brain matter. A clear ring around the scaring is visible with contrast enhancement. Symptoms are similar to normal Multiple Sclerosis. Tumefactive lesion may mimic a malignant tumour or a cerebral abscess resulting in complications during the diagnosis of Tumefactive MS.

**Neuromyelitis optica (NMO)** is another sub form of Multiple Sclerosis. It is called Devic's disease, after Eugene Devic who first described it in 1894. Although the first known case was documented by Sir Thomas Albutt in 1870 it was clearly defined by Eugene Devic. This type of multiple sclerosis only attacks the eyes and the spinal cord.

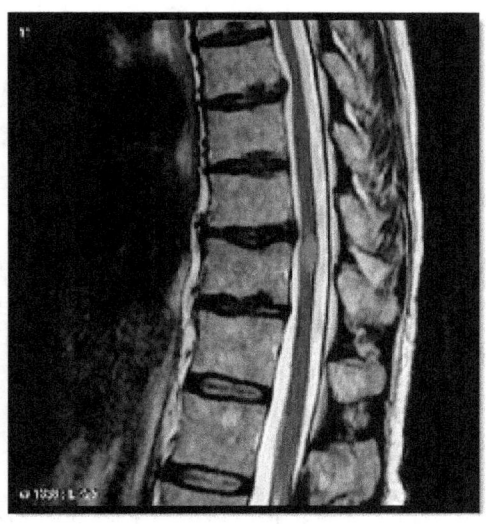

[21] Transverse Myelitis. (Image source: Wikipedia. Author: Frank Gaillard)

NMO normally is normally classified with optic neuritis in one or both eyes and severe weakness in the limbs. The inflammation can sometimes also affect the brain, but it is different from the way normal multiple sclerosis affects the brain. In normal multiple sclerosis, the T cells attacks the myelin sheath of the nerve, whereas with NMO this attack is by the antibody cells called the NMO-IgG. A simple spinal tap can indicate if these antibodies are present in the spinal fluid. Immunoglobulin G is present in most forms of Multiple Sclerosis, but different markers points to different forms of Multiple Sclerosis. NMO is characterized by transverse myelitis. Transverse Myelitis is the involvement of lesions in the spinal cord.

Treatment for NMO consists mainly of intravenous steroids. As a secondary measure, patients are also treated with immune suppressants. Unlike normal

Multiple Sclerosis, these patients are normally severely disabled after the first attack. Most patients also have permanent visual loss after the first attack. This type of multiple sclerosis is also referred to as transverse myelitis.

In 2006 the Mayo Clinic proposed a revised set of criteria for diagnosis of Devic's disease. The new guidelines require two absolute criteria plus at least two of three supportive criteria.

Absolute criteria:

- Optic neuritis

- Acute myelitis

Supportive criteria:

- Brain MRI not meeting criteria for MS at disease onset

- The presence of lesions in the spinal cord with T2-weighted signal extending over three or more vertebral segments, indicating a relatively large lesion in the spinal cord

- Definitive NMO-IgG markers in the spinal cord fluid.

Currently as with any form of Multiple Sclerosis, there is no cure and attacks are treated with short courses of high dosage intravenous corticosteroids.

Plasmapheresis is used if the patient does not respond to normal treatment. Ok; now I have the laymen confused. Plasmapheresis is as the Greek term defines it "The taking away and replacing of an item" and in this case, the plasma cells in blood. The dangerous NMO antibodies are removed from the blood by special filters and the blood replaced. The procedure is very similar to dialysis in kidney failure.

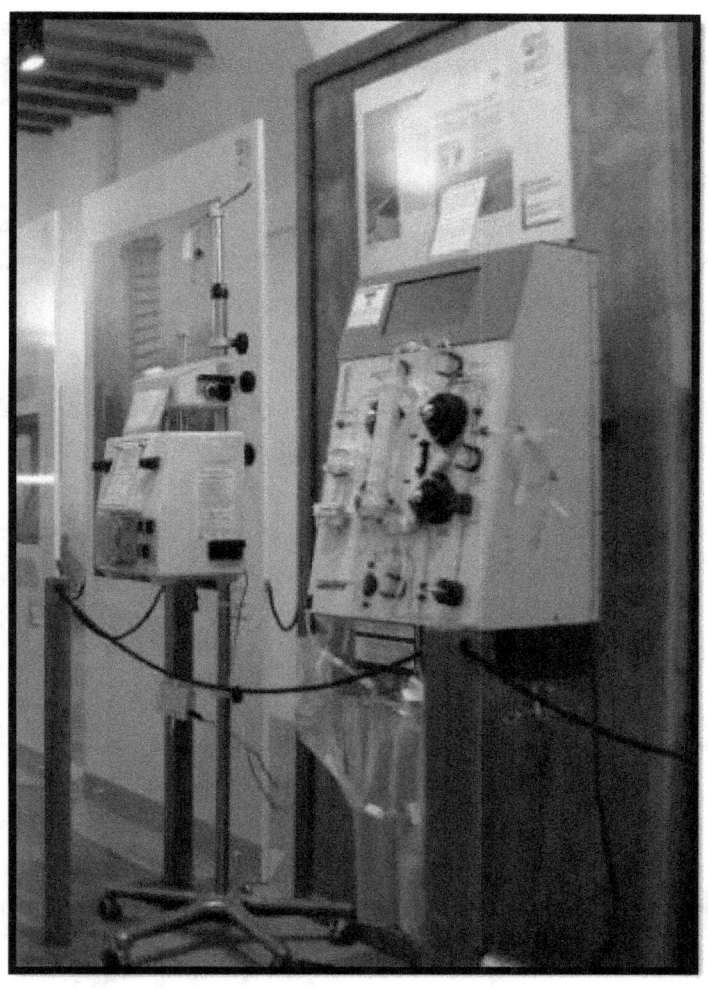

[22] Plasmapheresis equipment (Image source: Wikipedia. Author: Mr Vacchi)

As a secondary precaution, immune suppressant drugs are used to control the severity of attacks in NMO. Frequently used immunosuppressant treatments include azathioprine (Imuran) plus prednisone, mycophenolate mofetil plus prednisone, rituximab, mitoxantrone, intravenous immunoglobulin (IVIG), and cyclophosphamide. The jury is still out as to whether these treatments do actually work or not, with some neurologists opposing this theory.

**Balo Concentric Sclerosis (BCS)** or "encephalitis periaxialis concentricais" a borderline type of Multiple Sclerosis and similar to standard multiple sclerosis. The common belief was that the prognosis BCS is similar to Marburg's Multiple Sclerosis, but today it is known that patients with this type of Multiple Sclerosis can survive or even have spontaneous remissions. BCS is also found to be asymptomatic, in other words the disease is present but very little or no symptoms presenting themselves. BCS is common in the Chinese and Philippine populations. BCS attacks start very rapidly and the duration is normally spread over weeks to a couple of months.

Balo Concentric Sclerosis clinical course is normally similar to Primary Progressive Multiple Sclerosis, but the Relapse Remitting course has been indicated. Lesions are found in the white matter of the cerebral hemispheres, cerebellum, brainstem, spinal cord, and optical cortex. The primary symptoms of BCS are more cognitive dysfunction than actual motor skill dysfunction. Symptoms include headaches, aphasia, cognitive or behavioural dysfunction and seizures. In certain cases visual impairment and ataxia is reported. The Ataxia can include sensory loss as well as motor skill problems.

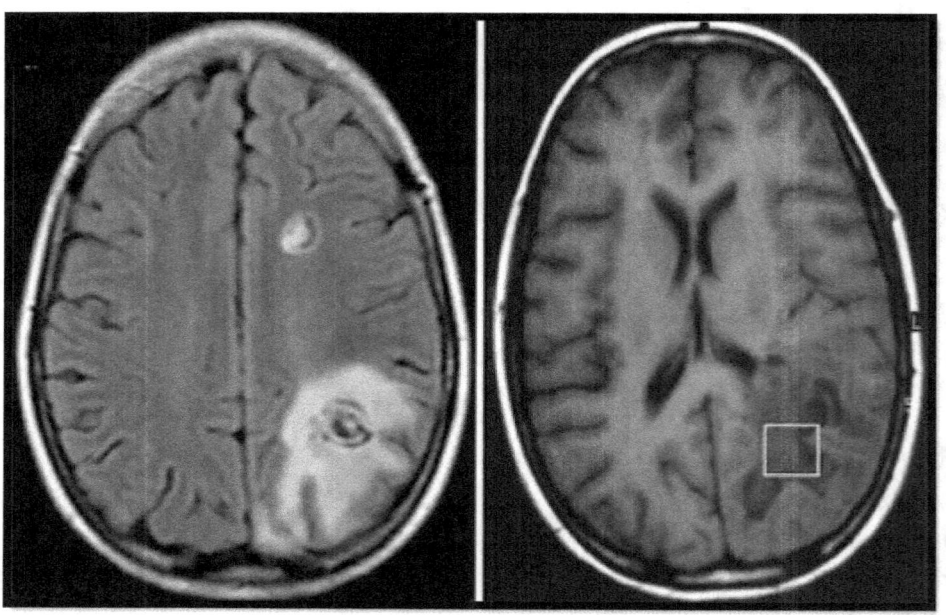

[23] Balo Concentric MRI image (Image source: National Library of Medicine (NLM))

Balo Concentric Sclerosis physical indicators in an MRI are concentric layers of demyelinated brain nerve tissue, usually accompanied by oligodendrocytes gliomas. Again a little elaboration is needed here. The term "concentric layers" stems from the fact that demyelination is concentrated around one centre point spreading out in layers, as compared to normal MS where the areas are more concentrated in spots. Oligodendrocytes are termed from the Greek word "brain cells with branches". Oligodendroglia is practically the glue structure that keeps the brain axons or nerves together. Gliomas are a type of tumor, indicating a mass, not cancerous, in Multiple Sclerosis.

Typical treatment is the use of corticosteroids, like in the case of normal MS. Indications are it responds to this treatment however cases have of spontaneous recovery has been reported.

# Different scales and criteria used to measure Multiple Sclerosis severity.

### Schumacher Criteria

The first criteria for diagnosing Multiple Sclerosis were adapted in 1965 by Dr Schumacher. This model is still used by some Neurologists today. The Schumacher criteria are outdated as most of modern diagnostic tools were not available back then. No MRI existed nor were Evoked Potential tests available as we have today, thus resulting in only clinical data being available with which to define Multiple Sclerosis. Schumacher proposed three classifications based in clinical observation: Clinically definite MS, probable MS and possible MS.

Six classical signs were used to determine Clinically Defined Multiple Sclerosis.

1.  Clinical signs of a problem in the CNS

2.  Evidence of two or more areas of CNS involvement

3.  Evidence of white matter involvement

4.  One of these: Two or more relapses (each lasting ≥ 24 hour and separated by at least 1 month) or progression (slow or stepwise)

5.  Patient should be between 10 and 50 year old at time of examination

6.  No better explanation for patient's symptoms and signs

The last clinical sign has and still is heavily criticised.

The Schumacher Criteria was replaced by the Poser Criteria in 1983. This was developed to include the advances of diagnostic techniques, namely the MRI scans and spinal taps that have helped neurologists to determine the existence of lesions and other clinical evidence to determine the diagnosis of Multiple Sclerosis.

The criteria can determine five conclusions:

1.  CDMS – Clinically definite MS. Needs two attacks and some clinical or clinical evidences

2. LSDMS – Laboratory supported definite MS, showing Oligoclonal bands and clinical or clinical evidences

3. CPMS – Clinically probable MS, with less restrict combinations.

4. LSPMS – Laboratory supported probable MS. Only two attacks is enough to enter this category

5. No MS – There is no clinical evidence of having MS.

Clinically definite MS

- 2 attacks and clinical evidence of 2 separate lesions

- 2 attacks, clinical evidence of one and paraclinical evidence of another separate lesion

Laboratory supported Definite MS

- 2 attacks, either clinical or paraclinical evidence of 1 lesion, and cerebrospinal fluid (CSF) immunologic abnormalities

- 1 attack, clinical evidence of 2 separate lesions & CSF abnormalities

- 1 attack, clinical evidence of 1 and paraclinical evidence of another separate lesion, and CSF abnormalities

Clinically probable MS

- 2 attacks and clinical evidence of 1 lesion

- 1 attack and clinical evidence of 2 separate lesions

- 1 attack, clinical evidence of 1 lesion, and paraclinical evidence of another separate lesion

Laboratory supported probable MS

- 2 attacks and CSF abnormalities

**Poser Criteria**

The Poser Criteria was more accurate, with post mortems indicating a diagnosis success rate of 84%. The advantage of the Poser diagnosis criteria for MS restricted doctors to normally diagnosis MS until a second attack takes place.

The McDonald criteria are named after neurologist W. Ian McDonald replaced the Poser Criteria in 2001. The McDonald criteria which were revised in 2005 with the advances in MRI and other tests that came onto the market.

1. Two or more relapses or attacks with two or more definite objective clinical lesions present. No additional tests were required if the clinical data is a definite indication of Multiple Sclerosis.

2. Two or more relapses with one definite objective clinical lesion present. This needs to be backed up with a flare up or dissemination in space on a MRI scan. Or a positive Cerebrospinal fluid test for immune abnormalities or more MRI lesions consisting with Multiple Sclerosis is ascertained.

3. One attack with two or more clinical objective lesions must be present. This needs to be backed up by with a flare-up or dissemination in time on a MRI or a second clinical attack.

4. One attack and one objective clinical lesion, with this type being a single symptomatic presentation. This needs to be backed up with a MRI with dissemination in space or a positive Cerebrospinal fluid test for immune abnormalities and two or more MRI lesions consistent with MS. Dissemination in time on a MRI or a second clinical attack. The word dissemination refers to scattering or in other words, scatters between lesions.

The positive indication of primary progressive Multiple Sclerosis is based on the following evaluation and information to back it up. A clear indication of 9 or more lesions on a MRI or four or more lesions on the MRI images with a positive VEP impairment results. There may also the presence of possibly two positive spinal cord lesions on a MRI images. A positive test for immune abnormalities in the cerebrospinal fluid

**McDonald Criteria**

The McDonald criterion is still in use today and was slightly revised in 2010. With more knowledge about the underlying pathology of MS being gathered, the concepts of subclinical, preclinical and CIS have been used together with the Poser original classification.

The Expanded Disability Status Scale is used to calculate the disability in Multiple Sclerosis scale, and is also used in clinical trials to mark the improvement or deterioration of the disease. The EDS scale is also used as a filter to determine patients for clinical trials, and to determine their Medications. It is a complicated calculation to determine the level of function loss in patient. Dr John Kurtzke in the 1950s was the first to develop a measurement to verify the disability status of people with Multiple Sclerosis, calling it the Disability Status Scale (DSS). This model has been modified over the last couple of decades and re- named to The Expanded Disability Status Scale or EDDS for short.

**EDDS is based on the following functional symptoms in Multiple Sclerosis patients:-**

1. The patient's ability to walk

2. The patient's coordination abilities.

3. The patient's speech and swallowing abilities.

4. The function of the patient's sensory and pain dysfunction.

5. The patient's bowel and bladder function.

6. The patient's visual status or impairment.

7. The patient's mental status.

8. Any other neurological functions.

**EDSS scoring in Multiple Sclerosis is done on the following criteria:-**

0.    Normal neurological exams.

1.0   One minimal functional system impairment with no disability

1.5   More than one functional system impairment with no disability.

2     One functional system impairment with limited disability.

2.5    One mild functional disability with one or two minimal functional system disability.

3.    Patient is fully mobile but has one moderate functional disability or three to four mild functional disabilities.

3.5. The patient is still fully mobile but has one moderate functional disability and mild disabilities in two functional systems, or the patient has two moderate functional system disabilities. More than five mild functional disabilities are also present.

4. The patient is fully mobile but has severe function system disabilities, although the patient can walk for 500 metres without aid. The patient can last for 12 hours without rest.

4.5. The patient is still fully mobile and up for the whole day. The patient could work the whole day but may need assistance and have some limitations. The patient can walk about 300 meters.

5. The patient can walk 200 meters without aid. The patient can still work but may not be able to work a full day. The patient needs more assistance at this stage.

5.5 The patient is restricted to walking about 100 meters without rest. The patient's full daily activities are restricted and he cannot work a full day.

6. The patient now requires a crutch or braces to walk 100 meters without rest. He is too severely disabled to do a full day's work.

6.5 The patient is mobile for about 20 meters with the help of crutches or support.

7.  The patient is restricted to a wheelchair. The patient can get in and out of a wheelchair without aid and can wheel around. The patient is still active for 12 hours a day. The patient can walk about 5 meters

7.5 The patient is restricted to a wheelchair and needs assistance getting in and out of it. He can wheel himself around but relies more on motorised wheelchairs for a full day's activity. He can only walk a few steps.

8. The patient is restricted to bed or a wheelchair. He cannot walk on his own. He can still stay active a full day in a wheelchair and still has most of the use of his arms. The patient can care for himself like bathing and eating.

8.5 The patient is now restricted to bed but still has the function of his arms and can still care for himself most of the times.

9.   The patient is still restricted to the bed but can still eat and talk. He needs assistance in all other matters.

9.5 The patient is totally restricted to bed, has difficulty talking and cannot feed himself and has difficulty swallowing.

10. Death due to Multiple sclerosis.

The problem with EDDS scoring is it may be a little out dated, with most of the scoring relying on the patient ability to walk. We know now that a lot of other function can influence Multiple Sclerosis patients. A good example is that the cognitive dysfunction in the patient could be higher than his mobile function which can lead to severe disability. Another factor is that with severe Optic Neuritis the patient could be nearly blind before his mobility is affected. Neuropathic pain can also lead to the patient being severely affected. As the patient relapses and recovers, his scoring on the EDS Scale can change with it.

**Fatigue Severity Scale (FSS)** is used to measure Fatigue in MS and is probably the one of the most common symptom in Multiple Sclerosis and has a daily impact on your life. It is also considered the one of the worst symptoms in multiple sclerosis and affects every person differently. Below is a table to calculate the severity of this symptom in Multiple Sclerosis. This model was adapted by the Consortium of Multiple Sclerosis Centres made up of 42 professionals in 1997.

1.   My motivation is lower when I am fatigued.

2.   Exercise brings on my fatigue.

3.   I am easily fatigued.

4.   Fatigue interferes with my physical functioning.

5.   Fatigue causes frequent problems for me

6.   My fatigue prevents sustained physical functioning.

7.   Fatigue interferes with carrying out certain duties and responsibilities.

8.   Fatigue is among my three most disabling symptoms.

9.  Fatigue interferes with my work, family, or social life.

The scoring is done by calculating the average response to the questions, adding it all up and dividing it by nine. Each symptom is scored on a range from 1-7 points. Multiple Sclerosis patients with depression alone score about 4 whilst patients with MS related fatigue score in the higher range. This is a very subjective measurement and is often over or under scored by patients. You need to be very objective when calculating this score, as lower values are normally very inconclusive and could be interpreted as a sign of depression.

# How does a typical Multiple Sclerosis attack start?

It has long been indicated that the first involvement of Multiple Sclerosis is the breakdown of the Blood Brain Barrier or BBB. The BBB is the special protection that our bodies have that prevents normal blood from entering the cerebrospinal fluid. This is the fluid that circulates in our brain ventricles and spinal cord or Central Nervous System (CNS). No blood ever enters the brain or spinal cord. Cells in this barrier lining carry metabolic products over the barrier to supply the brain with the necessary protein to survive. The BBB protects the brain from T-Cells or antibody cells from entering the brain. For reasons still largely unknown, a breakdown occurs in the BBB that causes antibody cells to enter the brain and start the body's own attack on the Myelin that protects our nerves or axons in the brain's white and grey matter. This breakdown causes small microscopic holes in the endothelium. The endothelium is a condensed pack cell lining in the veins that prevents blood from passing through the veins or arteries. I will elaborate more on this a bit later.

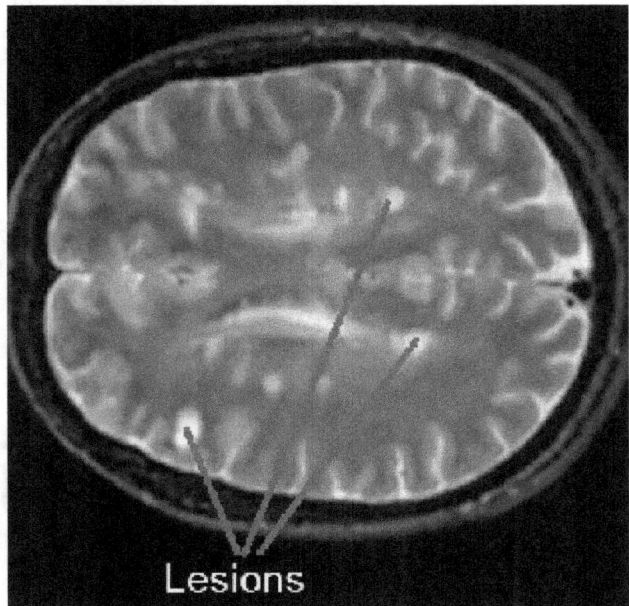

[24] Typical Multiple Sclerosis attack with blue marks showing lesions (Image courtesy of anonymous patient)

This process starts with the breakdown of the blood brain barrier. With the breakdown of this barrier antibodies are able to travel to the CNS. When these antibodies reach the CNS, it attacks the nerve axon of the CNS. This leads to the fatty sheath being stripped down over these axons, causing what is called demyelination. The cells that attack the CNS are called T helper cells. In a Multiple Sclerosis patient these helper cells cannot distinguish normal own CNS parts and foreign parts. The helper cells attack the normal parts of the CNS, seeing it as a foreign invader and attacking it as such to try to get rid of this virus. The inflammation process then starts and the body produces more antibodies and immune cells to help fight this virus. This is when the immune system goes into overdrive and attacks the nerves fatty tissue and strips this fatty sheath off the axons.

In these attacks, the axon can also be damaged and the brain tries to compensate for this damage. However, eventually these attacks lead to permanent axonal damage eventually leading to breaks in the axons which are not repairable. Multiple Sclerosis symptoms appear as a result of these lesions caused by a demyelination attack. Because the attacks take place in different parts of the CNS, the symptoms will vary drastically from patient to patient. After each attack the sheath is damaged and a process of re-myelination begins. Unfortunately with each attack the sheath is repaired to a thinner than usual extent. Every attack there after leaves the nerve with less and less Myelin. When the sheath is stripped down to such an extent that it cannot be repaired, a scar like plague is built up around the nerve. This multiple scaring is what is referred to as Multiple Sclerosis.

In a typical Flare up Gadolinium, a contrast agent given intravenously will highlight active lesion, by showing up more white on the MRI scan.

There are various other factors that also play a vital role in Multiple Sclerosis attack, but the above is a typical attack in a nutshell. After a typical Flare up the blood brain barrier regains its integrity, and some T-cells remain trapped in the brain.

**The Function of CSF in the brain.**

Now here is where a lot of elaboration is required. As I already mentioned, your brain and spinal has no blood in it what so ever, but is surrounded and floats in Cerebral Spinal Fluid. The medical term is Cerebrospinal Fluid or CSF for short. It is a clear colourless fluid and is produce in the choroid plexus. Choroid plexus is coined from Greek "khorion" - "membrane enclosing the foetus or afterbirth" and "plexus" from Latin "braid or network". There are four Choroid Plexi (plural for plexus) located in the brain. The CSF is recycled 4 times per day in order to clean out metabolites from the brain. The choroid plexus must produce about 500 millilitres of CSF fluid daily. Like blood the CSF also pulsates in the brain.

The system comprises four ventricles:

- Right and left lateral ventricles (the first and second ventricles)
- Third ventricle
- Fourth ventricle

The CSF in the brain acts as a cushion or buffer for the cortex, providing a basic mechanical and immunological protection to the brain inside the skull and serves a vital function in cerebral auto regulation of cerebral blood flow. Each system has blood vessels running in them. The transfer of proteins, nutrients and oxygen etc. is achieved by these elements crossing the blood brain barrier.

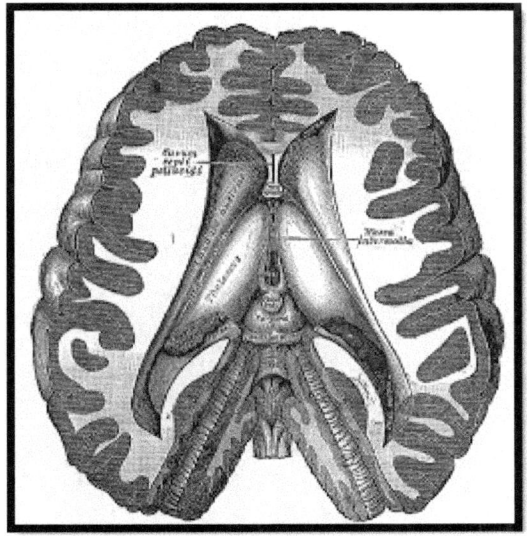

[25] The ventricles of the brain.

The CSF has several functions including:

1.  Protection: the CSF protects the brain from damage by "buffering" the brain. In other words, the CSF acts to cushion a blow to the head and lessen the impact.
2.  Buoyancy: because the brain is immersed in fluid, the net weight of the brain is reduced from about 1,400 gm. to about 25 gm. Therefore, pressure at the base of the brain is reduced.
3.  Excretion of waste products: the one-way flow from the CSF to the blood takes potentially harmful metabolites, drugs and other substances away from the brain.
4.  Endocrine medium for the brain: the CSF serves to transport hormones to other areas of the brain. Hormones released into the CSF can be carried to remote sites of the brain where they may act.

The IgG index is a clear indicator of Multiple Sclerosis in CSF. Immunoglobulin G (IgG) is an antibody isotype. IgG is the main antibody isotype found in blood and extracellular fluid allowing it to control infection of body tissues. This index is measured calculating the index of IgG anti bodies in the cerebral fluid.

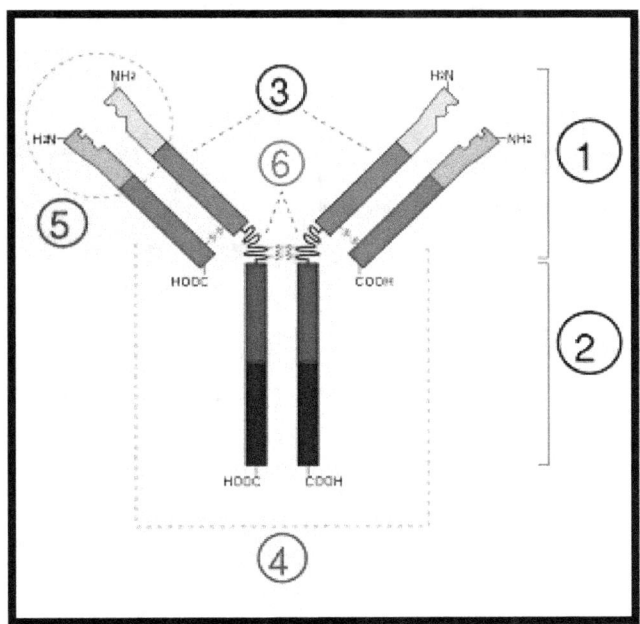

[26] Immunoglobulin G (Image source: Wikipedia. Author: Y_tambe)

Arachnoid granulations are small protrusions of the arachnoid, the thin second layer covering the brain, in the Dura mater or, in other words, the thick outer layer. They protrude into the venous sinuses of the brain, and allow cerebrospinal fluid (CSF) to exit the brain and enter the blood stream. CSF flows down the spinal cord to the "Cauda equine" which is a bundle of nerve roots stemming from the lumbar enlargement and "conus medullaris"; the end point of the spinal cord. This is the location where a spinal tap is normally performed.

Now this sounds all very complex and to the layman it certainly is, but in order to explain the effects of a Multiple Sclerosis attack, this chapter is an essential element.

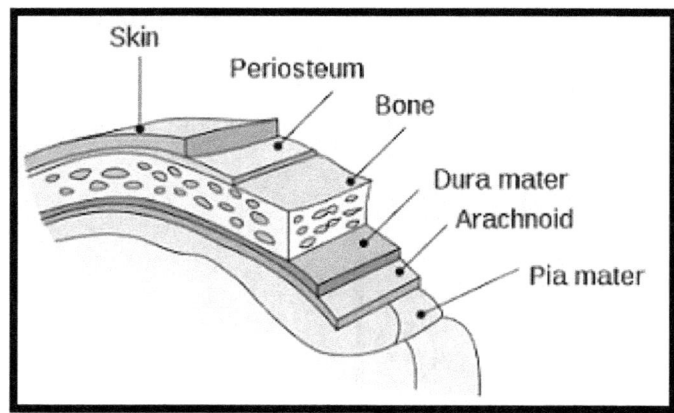

[27] Outer Layer of the skull protecting the brain (Image source: Wikipedia. Credit: National Institutes of Health)

In a typical Multiple Sclerosis relapse or onset, the theory is that the blood brain barrier fails, be it by a virus or other factors. The exact reason it fails is still not completely understood. Some suggestions are genetic factors playing a role in the blood brain barrier make-up whilst others point to a virus. There are also indications that the blood brain barrier opens up to let T-Killer cells in to fight an infection or inflammation in the brain. There are also suggestions that the BBB fails due to increased blood vessels strain.

There has always been a clear link between Multiple Sclerosis and the ventricle system in the brain. The earliest studies of MS brains clearly indicate the lesions to form from the ventricles outwards. The lesions around the ventricle was named "Dawson's Fingers" named after James Walker Dawson (1870, India - 26 June 1927, Edinburgh) who was a Scottish pathologist remembered for his work on Multiple Sclerosis including the description Dawson's fingers. Dawson's fingers spread along, and from, large periventricular collecting veins, and are attributed to inflammation around a vein in the MS brain.

In 1931 Gabriel Steiner, at the University of Heidelberg, drew vivid pictures of the spread of Multiple Sclerosis into the cerebral hemispheres. Apart from presenting schematic drawings of process-typical intrusions into the cerebral cortex from its outer side, he impressively illustrated the specific plaques' bumpy, stalked or splashy projections off the ventricular borders. Because the lesion formations preferentially burst forth at the lateral cerebral ventricles' outer angles, this site was referred to by the telling German name "Wetterwinkel", denoting a source of thunderstorms and deluges. This site has also come to be known as "Steiner's Wetterwinkel". All in all, Steiner's pictures lucidly highlighted what Dawson's description of cerebral Multiple Sclerosis had disclosed fifteen years before.

In 1962 Steiner, then at Wayne State University, demonstrated again that cerebral Multiple Sclerosis is primarily characterized by smooth, rounded or peaked lesions rising off of the ventricular border. Besides showing that ventricle-based lesion "tongues" can also connect with more peripheral plaques, Steiner now observed that isolated, ovoid or spherical lesion "splashes" also arise from blood-vessels far away from the ventricles. Such separate plaques are referred to here as "Steiner's splashes".

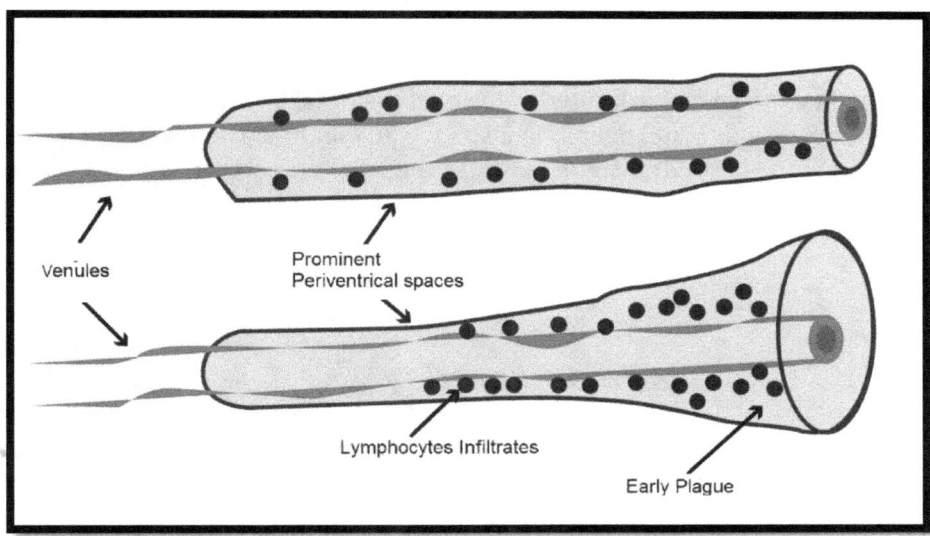

[28] Illustration of perivenular inflammatory infiltrates that cause lesion formation and enlarged perivenular spaces in Multiple Sclerosis. The prominent perivenular spaces can be with (bottom vessel) or without (top vessel) lesion association. (Image courtesy of Grant Groenenstein)

Dawson fingers are easily seen on RMI scans in Multiple Sclerosis, especially in those with severe Multiple Sclerosis. The condition is thought to be the result of inflammation or mechanical damage by blood pressure around the long axis of medullary veins in the brain or spinal cord. Demyelination begins with the blood–

brain barrier breakdown. There is a tight vascular barrier between the blood and brain that should prevent the passage of antibodies through it, but in MS patients, it does not function. For unknown reasons, special areas appear in the brain and spine, followed by leaks in the blood–brain barrier where immune cells infiltrate.

In Multiple Sclerosis, cells of the immune system infiltrate the brain tissue, where they cause damage. The process as to how the cells break through the blood brain barrier was never fully understood. Until now, the sole evidence that the immune cells really do manage to reach the nerve cells is the presence of immune cells in brain tissue samples. In 2009, a team of scientists from the Max Planck Institute of Neurobiology, the University Medical Centre Göttingen, and other institutes, demonstrated the movements of these cells under the microscope for the very first time. In the process, they discovered several new behavioural traits of the immune cells. Their consolidated findings mark a significant step forward in our understanding of this complex disease.

Below is the first image ever captured in mice, of the breakdown in the Blood Brain Barrier. This image was taken over a time span of 20 minutes. The red indicate the blood vessels in the brain. The green indicates the T-cells breach of the blood brain barrier and spread into the brain tissue.

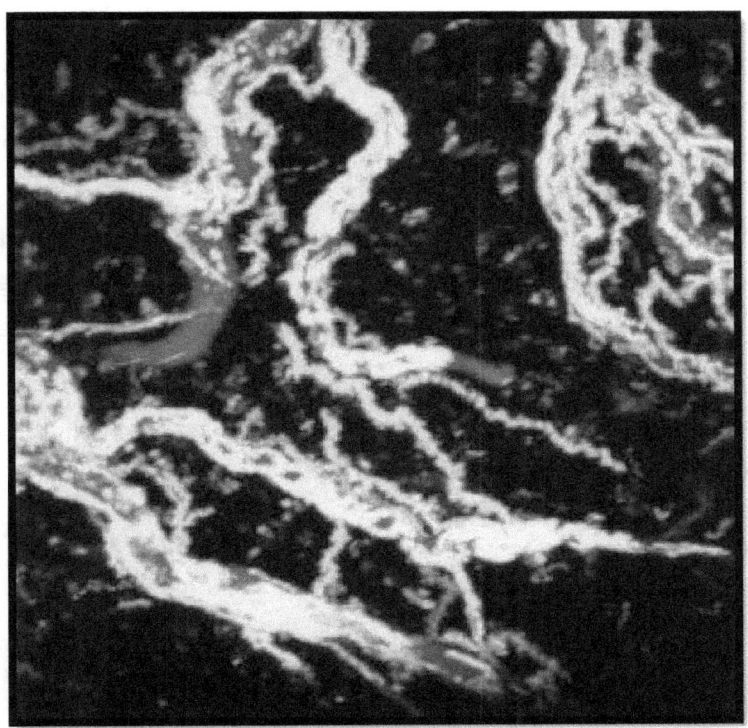

[29] Blood brain barrier breach (Image credit: Max Planck Institute of Neurobiology / Bartholomäus)

Using a two-photon microscope, the researchers succeeded in tracing the movements of aggressive T-cells labelled with the green fluorescent protein (GFP) in the living tissue of rats and demonstrated the movement of these cells into the brain. Outside the nervous system the cells moved as they should, only clinging to the blood vessel walls every once in a while. However once they reached the nervous system these cells acted very differently. Here the cells actually cling to the walls and even started creeping against the actual blood flow. Then the cells broke through the vessel walls entering the brain and searching for new pathways. It was thus only a question of time before the T-cells encountered one of the phagocytic cells abundant on the outer linings of blood vessels and on the surface of the nerve tissue. When a mobile T-cell came across such a phagocyte, the two cells formed a closely connected pair. Some of these pairs remained inseparable for several minutes.

As suspected, once paired with the phagocyte they started their attack on the nervous system. However, also noted was that some of the anti-bodies used to treat Multiple Sclerosis stop them from creeping. Up until now, it was believed that these anti-bodies prevent the breach in the blood brain barrier, but this new insight shows it actually prevents them from creeping.

This all being said we must take note that the blood brain barrier does get breached in other diseases as well, and we cannot conclude that this may not be the only reason we develop Multiple Sclerosis. These lead researchers to believe there may be a virus, or genetics involved.

There are some other factors in play as well. This is the grey area of Multiple Sclerosis. And I will touch on them in the next chapter.

# Possible causes of Multiple Sclerosis.

**Epstein Barr virus** or EBV for short has been indicated as a possible trigger of Multiple Sclerosis. It is a known fact in the medical world that nearly 95% of all the people under the age of 40 have antibodies to EBV in their systems. However it is estimated that we all have been exposed to EBV before the age of 20. Now to find out how EBV can cause MS, we need to look more deeply in the makeup of EBV and how it affects us.

EBV or glandular fever is caused by the human herpes virus 4(HH4 for short). It is also known as mononucleosis. It is one of the most common viruses that affects the human body. As a child, when you do come into contact with EBV, you may be symptom free, or you may suffer mild to severe symptoms which include fever and swollen glands. In some cases it may only present itself as a cold sore, with or without fever. It is also called the "kissing disease" because it remains in the immune system and dormant in the throat, and is normally spread by a simple kiss. Some forms of recurring tonsillitis and mumps that extend passed their normal period, is also an indication of EBV. And in some rare cases of measles, also tie in with EBV although this is still to be confirmed. Another clear case of EBV is regular throat infections, irritating but not enough to send you to the doctors.

Infectious mononucleosis can also affect the spleen and liver, causing them to swell. Heart problems and ventricle involvement is also indicated in some cases of EBV. In severe cases of EBV the Central Nervous System is also involved. Certain studies are also being done to see if Chronic Fatigue Syndrome (CSF) is caused by mononucleosis.

A Multiple Sclerosis patient has a higher count of T-cells that protect the body against EBV. The problem comes in with the make-up of these EBV antibodies that is present in a MS Patient. The "epitope" protein or the micromolucule that is recognised by the anti-EBV killer T-cells of the immune system is similar to the protein "epitope" make up of Myelin. So in laymen's terms, the same protein make up of EBV is similar to the make-up of the protein of Myelin protein. The T-Cells can't distinguish between the two and therefore it summons helper cells or B-Cells to attack the Myelin in a MS patient. Normally the body will stop such a self-attack, but it seems that the Myelin Oligodendrocytes Glycoproteins (MOG) is not protected by the body, in a MS patient. The theory behind this is the Vitamin-D responsive switch may be involved in this process.

A recent study that was done in Canada on children that have Multiple Sclerosis has indicated that 83% of children with MS have the EBV virus in their system, while in the control group of healthy children only 43% had the EBV virus in their system. Further studies also indicate a 96% of EBV anti bodies in adults with MS although this is still to be confirmed)

Further evidence to this, are the studies where mice are injected with the protein that makes up Myelin, the same reaction does take place. They basically replicate Multiple Sclerosis in mice by a process called experimental autoimmune encephalomyelitis, or EAE for short.

Now to start when we get infected with EBV, somewhere in our growing up years or at a later stage in life, it may be in the form of a latent infection, in other words, we don't even know we are infected with it. We either show little or no sign of any infections, or it can be in the form of Glandular Fewer or Mononucleosis and even tonsillitis. However it is now documented that about 96% of adults have the EBV antibodies in their system.

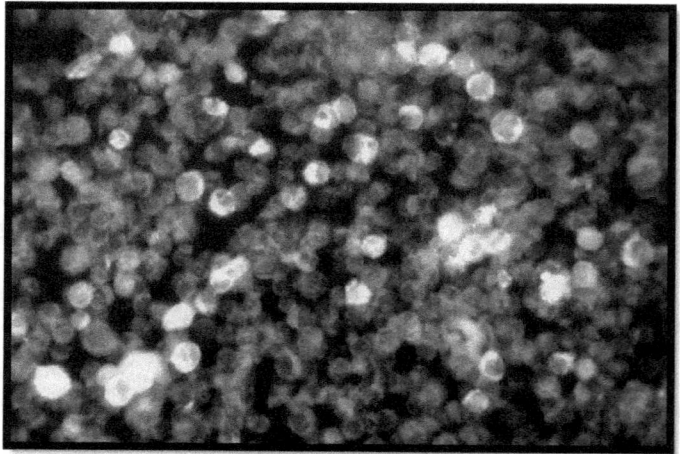

[30] Epstein Barr virus using a FA staining technique (Image Source: CDC/Dr. Paul M. Feorino)

However recent studies has shown that in adults with Multiple Sclerosis, the level of antibodies to EBV is 99%, compared to the control group where this level is only

90-95%. In other words 99% of all adults with MS have EBV antibodies in their system. Also the study of children with MS has shown that up to 99% have the EBV antibodies in their system compared to the control group of healthy children with only 43%. This strongly suggests that we need to be infected with EBV before we can actually develop Multiple Sclerosis. Now with the case of infectious mononucleosis or infectious glandular fewer the EBV antibody levels are lot higher than in the case of non-infectious mononucleosis. EBV anti bodies have been found in MS patients 20 years before the onset of Multiple Sclerosis. Also the spinal fluid of a Multiple Sclerosis patient has shown an immune response to EBV, in other words, there are antibodies in the spinal fluid to EBV. However due to the absence of any studies of EBV in the brain, this could never be confirmed. This is partly due to poor preservation of MS brains and not the correct diagnostic material available at the time.

But they took it on step further and decided to study the brain of MS patients as well, to see if the presence of EBV antibodies can also be found in the brain. We know that there are immune responses in the brain, as the inflammation process is clearly visible on an MRI (Flare up spots on the MRI). But what causes this immune response? They did autopsies on the brain tissues of MS patients to see whether there are latent EBV infections in the brain, or if there are any antibodies in the MS brain. Now the findings of these studies were astounding.

In all the cases, they found that there are definitely antibodies to the EBV virus. Because the protein make up of EBV is similar to the protein make-up of Myelin, it would be natural to see that the areas of demyelination appear close to where there is an EBV anti-body built up in the brain. The study did prove that. In the areas of the brain where there was a large collection of EBV anti-bodies, the MS lesion load was far more active. Now we know that MS is caused by an immune response, in other words, our own antibodies do attack our Central Nervous system. In all of the areas of inflammation that they have studied in the brain, they found a large presence of B-cells. B-cells are the helper cell that our bodies call up to defend our body against any infections. They also tested to exclude the possibility of other infection, or whether this is the case in a control group. They could however not find any of the indication of the above process in the control group autopsies. So in conclusion, they found that in the areas of the brain where there are EBV anti bodies present, there was an MS lesion load and a B-cell presence.

Further to this it is now also clear why a very bad case of Glandular Fewer or Mononucleosis can have the same symptoms as early Multiple Sclerosis. As the immune response to a major EBV infection can cause the same symptoms as the immune response that starts Multiple Sclerosis.

Based on the above studies they are currently expanding this research to include the role that EBV plays in the development of Multiple Sclerosis and other auto immune responsive disease like Rheumatoid Arthritis. However, the question that still needs to be answered fully is what role does the blood brain barrier play in protecting the brain from this type of reaction, or whether EBV can actually cause blood brain barrier breakdown? Also further studies need to be done to see if the immune attack is due to the inflammation process of MS, or whether the attack is in response to a re-activation of an EBV infection in the brain.

To this day there is no cure, or treatment for EBV. Treatment is symptomatic and rest. Currently there is also no vaccine for EBV. Once exposed to EBV it remains latent for the most part your life in your throat and blood and you may have reactivation of EBV without any clinical signs.

**Vitamin D deficiency and Multiple Sclerosis** has a clear link that has been researched over many years. Now before I can explain that link, I must first explain Vitamin D and how the body deals with it. Most forms of Vitamin D are a secosteroid responsible for intestinal absorption of calcium and phosphate. This is a steroid with a broken binding in its rings. The two forms that we are interested in are Vitamin D2 and D3. Vitamin D2 is found in fish, plants and fungus. It gets manufactured when the above comes in contact with UV rays in sunlight. Humans do not manufacture Vitamin D2.

Vitamin D3 is manufactured in humans when the skin comes into contact with the ultra violet (UV) rays in sunlight. This production of Vitamin D only takes place when the UV index is greater than 3. At the equator, the UV index is always greater than 3. The further away you go from the equator the lower the UV index becomes. In normal seasonal climates, when there are seasonal changes, this UV index is only achieved in the spring, summer and fall. The closer you move to the arctic, this UV index is never that high. In some climates this index is only achieved in the summer i.e. United Kingdom. A 15 min - 30 min exposure to sunlight on the arms and face is enough to create your daily requirement of D3. Any longer exposure to Vitamin D will only breakdown and degrade as fast as it was created. Another factor in this is the skin natural light filter. This is called Melanin, and the greater the content of melanin, the longer the exposure needs to be.

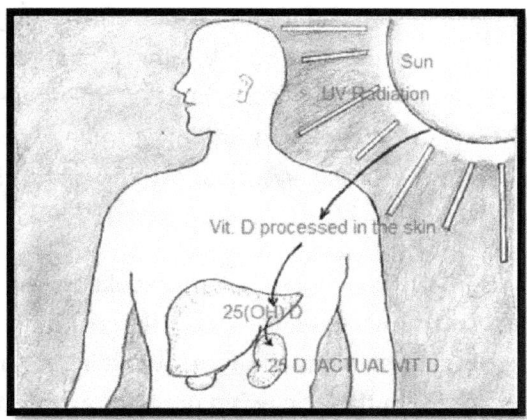

[31] Vitamin D manufacturing process in the body. (Image courtesy of Claudette Ann Groenenstein)

When Vitamin D2 is absorbed in foods, or D3 is created in the skin it travels to the liver and kidneys to form Dihydroxyvitamin D or 1,25D. This is the vitamin D in hormone form that we need. Vitamin D deficiency can be as a result of not enough intake in your diet, or under-exposure to sunlight.  Further causes can be a malfunction in the kidneys and the liver. Other factors can also be skin fat or skin tone.

No diet alone can give you enough Vitamin D for your daily requirement. A high fish diet can help to produce enough Vitamin D, but it still falls short of daily requirements.

Certain theories and studies suggest that Vitamin D is the one aspect that you need in childhood if you are genetically inclined to develop Multiple Sclerosis. We have a switch in the gene system called the Vitamin D responsive switch. This switch in our gene system is responsible for the body's immune system to ascertain what normal proteins in the body are and what a foreign invader is. If a person with a Vitamin D responsive form of this switch did not get enough Vitamin D in childhood, this switch is not activated properly. This may cause the body to attack itself in Multiple

Sclerosis patients later in life. Based on this theory and certain studies, scientists recommend that it may even be important for pregnant mothers to receive Vitamin D, so as to prevent the infant from developing MS.

There is also an indication that taking Vitamin D if you have Multiple Sclerosis may slow down the progress of the disease. This is still a theory and is currently being studied. It does not suggest taking Vitamin D or being on a high Vitamin D diet can cure this disease. It may certainly help to slow down the disease, but this still needs verification. A clinical trial sponsored by Charite University in Berlin, Germany was begun in 2011, with the goal of examining the efficacy, safety and tolerability of Vitamin D3 in the treatment of Multiple Sclerosis.

**Geographical influences on Multiple Sclerosis** have long been speculated and documented that Vitamin D deficiency could increase the risk of developing Multiple Sclerosis. The more we are exposed to sunlight the more vitamin D our bodies produce. Vitamin D is produced primarily in the skin, when you are exposed to Ultraviolet rays.

Studies show that the further away you are from the Equator, the more likely the tendency to develop Multiple Sclerosis. So areas like Canada, the Northern US and Northern Europe has the highest population of Multiple Sclerosis Sufferers. The next on the list are Russia, South East Europe and South West Europe. Following them are Central US, South Europe and South Australia and finally Southern US, Southern Africa, Northern Australia and Far North Africa. However, there are important exceptions to the north–south pattern and changes in prevalence rates over time, in general, this trend might be disappearing.

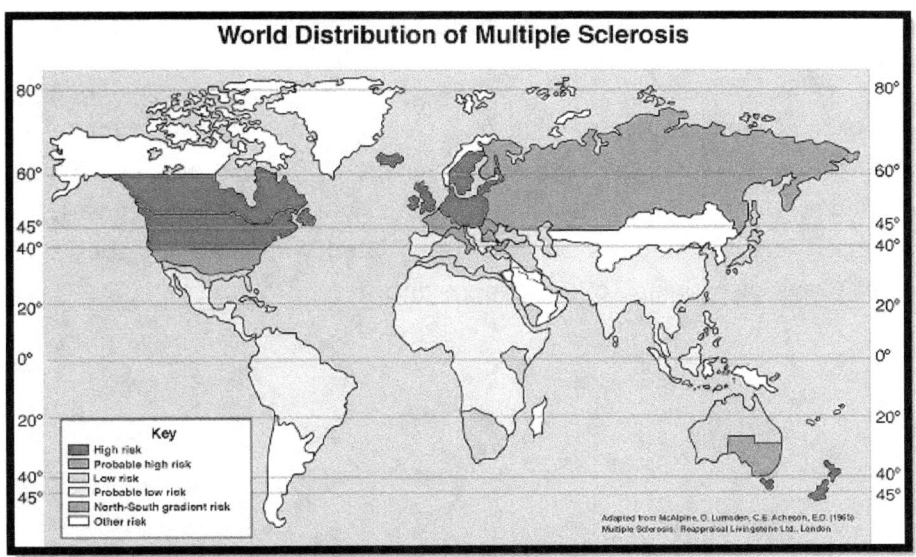

[32] Distribution of Multiple Sclerosis

Multiple Sclerosis has a prevalence that ranges between 2 and 150 per 100,000 depending on the country or specific population. Environmental factors during childhood may play an important role in the development of MS later in life. Several studies of migrants show that if migration occurs before the age of 15, the migrant acquires the new region's susceptibility to MS. If migration takes place after age 15, the migrant retains the susceptibility of his home country. Your month of birth can also affect MS, with fewer patients born in November being diagnosed with MS later in life, than those born in May.

Now with all of the above you would think that when you have Multiple Sclerosis, sunlight would be good for you. In fact, it is totally the opposite because sunlight and heat can exacerbate the effects of Multiple Sclerosis as explained in the Uhtoff's Phenomenon.

**Genetics** has been indicated in Multiple Sclerosis for some time now. A recent study found a new genetic risk factor for Multiple Sclerosis patients who have certain variations or mutations of two different genes; IL7RA and IL2RA and are more likely to have MS than the normal population. IZ7RA and IL2RA are proteins that guide the actions of one type of the immune system's killer T-Cells. As genes control how proteins are made up in the body, changes in protein type represent a difference in your genetic make-up.

The MS version of the protein may contribute to MS by guiding those immune cells to attack the Central Nervous System, which leads to demyelination and lesions on the brain and spinal cord. The demyelination and lesions causes the huge variety of MS symptoms. IL2R mutations have been associated with type 1 diabetes and Myasthenia Gravis disease, and other immune disorders.

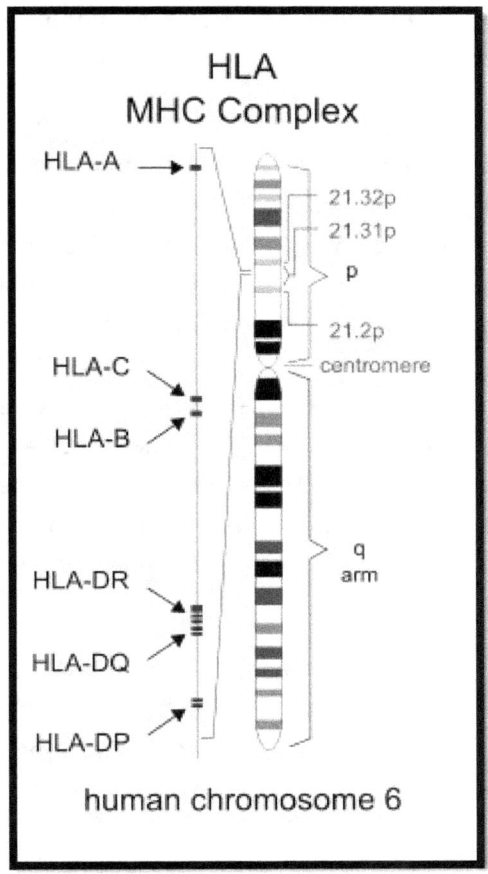

[33] Human Chromosome 6 Genetic code (Image source: Wikipedia. Author: Pdeitiker)

The gene mutation does not lead to MS but instead, because of a direct causal link, these genes could increase susceptibility to MS, meaning that other factors are still at work. This just means that certain people with these genes are 20 to 30% more likely to have MS. If the overall risk of MS is 1 in 1000, and you have these genes, your risk becomes 1 in 770.

Multiple Sclerosis diagnosis is higher in relatives of a person with the disease than in the general population, especially in the case of siblings, parents, and children. The disease has an overall increase rate of 20% if a relative has/had MS. In the case of identical twins, it occurs only in about 35% of cases, while it goes down to around 5% in the case of siblings and even lower in half-siblings. This indicates susceptibility is partly genically driven. Multiple Sclerosis seems to be more common in some ethnic groups than others.

"Apart from familial studies, specific genes have been linked with MS. Differences in the human leukocyte antigen (HLA) system—a group of genes in chromosome 6 that serves as the major histocompatibility complex (MHC) in humans—increase the probability of suffering MS. The most consistent finding is the association between Multiple Sclerosis and mutation types of the MHC defined as DR15 and DQ6. Other "loci" or the specific location of a gene or DNA sequence on a chromosome have shown a protective effect, such as HLA-C554 and HLA-DRB1*11". Major histocompatibility complex (MHC) is a cell surface molecule encoded by a large gene family in all vertebrates. MHC molecules mediate interactions of leukocytes, also called white blood cells (WBCs), which are immune cells, with other leukocytes or body cells. Differences in this genetic make-up can be an attributing factor to the Killer T-Cells going hay-wire and attacking our own body.

Further understanding the MS disease process may generate new ideas for treatment. These genes cause a defect in certain proteins which regulate immune system attack on our body. Essentially, if we could repair these proteins or repair their actions, we may be able to stop the Killer T-cells from attacking our Myelin sheath.

Scientists are looking into genetics as a future prevention or gene therapy for Multiple Sclerosis.

**Trauma** has been stated throughout history as a possible cause of Multiple Sclerosis. MS patients frequently relate the onset of the disease or exacerbation of symptoms to a traumatic episode or event in their lives. This could be a physical injury such as a blow to the head with concussion, a vehicle accident, or an excessive stress such as marriage failures or grief over the loss of a loved one. This theory has been debunked through history, by various trials and studies. Only one case was ever taken to court and won, only to be overthrown in the Court of Appeals.

It is however true, that undue stress can cause your symptoms to worsen and a flare up to last longer than normal to a certain extent. And as with any diseases, stressful situations should be avoided as it can have an impact on recovery. Remember the golden rule "A healthy mind supports a healthy body".

There is however the exception that a heavy electrical shock could lead to the onset of MS, with a couple of possible cases noted trough history.

# Other Possible causes of Multiple Sclerosis

**Multiple Sclerosis; does it have a vascular connection?**

Since the dawn of Multiple Sclerosis (MS) there have been suggestions that MS may have a vascular link. This link has been repeatedly suggested over the last 160 years of Multiple Sclerosis. In fact, the earliest suggestion was in 1848 before the name MS was even known. The first documented case was published by a German pathologist by the name of Rindfleisch. In 1863 five years before Charcot first describe Multiple Sclerosis and naming this disease, Rindfleisch described pathological findings from autopsies he did on patients that had died from this strange disease.

Dr Charcot first described that there was a strong link between the major veins and the brain, as these lesions tend to form more frequently near the major arteries in the brain. This was also described by Dr James Walker Dawson in 1916, in which he described how these lesions run from the brain lateral ventricles in finger like, dome or cone shapes lesions. In 1931 Gabriel Steiner produced the first sketches indicating that these lesions run from the ventricles outwards.

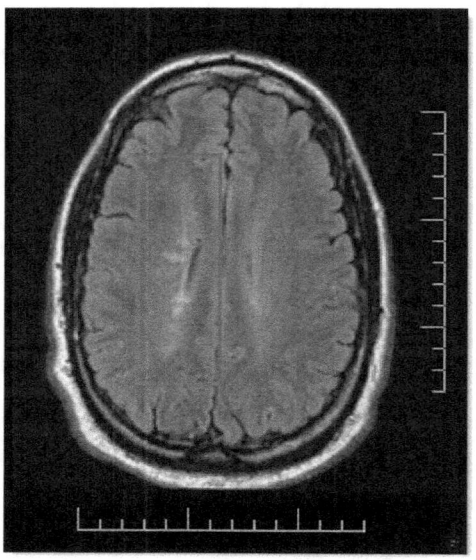

[34] Dawson Fingers on a modern MRI scan (Image source: Wikipedia. Author: VoiceOfReason)

He published that the altered parts of the white matter seem to have a red point in the middle of each individual lesion. He noted small vessels engorged with blood at these focal points. But he also noted that all these vessel structures seemed to be intact but seemed to have a characteristic indication of inflammation. He therefore speculated that an inflammation of the blood vessels played a role in what we today call Multiple Sclerosis. However no clear link could be found between this unique characteristic effect on the blood vessels and Multiple Sclerosis. This theory was also demonstrated by many other publications in the history of Multiple sclerosis.

In 1937 Tracey Putman and Alexandra Adler specifically described that cerebral plaques or lesions developed closely to the large epiventrical veins in the brain. They also demonstrated distortions on the veins near the lesion area. Putman indicated this link in Multiple Sclerosis in the 1930s, and even tried to replicate this in dogs. This replication was done by injecting obstructing agents in the longitudinal sinus veins of dogs. The obstructing agents consisted of lard oil. The lesions that were demonstrated after this experiment were similar to Multiple Sclerosis, although not exactly, being that it resembled more the damage caused by a mini stroke than Multiple Sclerosis. Also noted was that the animal model, indicated Multiple Sclerosis as an immune response, and formed a better picture than Putman's experiments.

The first treatment of MS as a vascular disease was done during 1939-1960. During this stage the first anti-coagulants or blood thinners were used to treat Multiple Sclerosis. The results of that era, although not widely published, indicated that there is some benefits for a Multiple Sclerosis patient, but this was relatively small and did not necessary slow down the disease. It did have an impact on the patient's progression to remission after the treatment. However this was never a controlled study, but the treatment was used as it did show immediate benefit to the relapse symptoms. The long term effects on Multiple Sclerosis was never fully addressed or studied but the outcome, based on patient records and doctor's experience, was that there were no long term benefits. The short term benefits were just that; very short term and were basically only symptomatic relief as such. So in came the next era and the treatment of MS with high dose steroids.

Brickner's stenosis was describe in 1950 and published, under what he called Transient sudden mini attacks of Multiple Sclerosis. He studied the blood vessels in the eyes of Multiple Sclerosis patients who complained of sudden blindness or vision loss. What he found was that MS patients showed signs of retinal arteriolar constrictions. He found that treatment with rapid acting vasodilation drugs showed a marked improvement in these patients visual acuity. Also noted was the fact that these constrictions disappeared by themselves and the visual acuity also increased. He also went on to demonstrate that a hot bath or shower can increase this phenomenon. Immediately after the increase of the body's core temperature, the phenomenon of retinal arteriolar constrictions was noted. Based on this findings he hypothesized that certain remission in MS can be attributed to spontaneous vasoconstriction disappearing. Further to this he also suggested that if this can happen in the eye it may also happen in other parts of the cerebral vascular system. In other words, he suggested that MS could be the result of constriction in certain veins in the brain. His theory has never been investigated fully.

Doctor Roy L. Swank (1909-2008), another well-known figure in the MS world, wrote a book on vasoconstrictions attributing this fact to thrombosis of the cerebral vascular system. His theory was based on the fact that certain foods can cause thrombosis in the cerebral vascular venous system and by following the right diet you could reduce the symptoms of Multiple Sclerosis. The Swank diet was introduced in 1948 and is still followed today by many MS Patients worldwide. The success of his diet has never been fully studied, although there is mixed reaction to his diet, with a few patients claiming that this diet has cured them. And then there is, of course, the opposite with the majority of patients reporting no or little benefit from this diet.

In the 1960s Dr Torben Fog, a Danish professor noted that MS lesions are predominantly around the small veins. He investigated the link between Multiple Sclerosis lesions and their direct relation to the veins. Fog could demonstrate that the lesions are in direct relation to the parent vein or the collecting vein in the brain. He indicated that the lesions first emerge close to the large veins collecting the blood from the brain. He stated that these veins are normally twisted and bended in an abnormal fashion. He also indicated that although the bulk of the lesions found near a vein have no direct relation to the vein size itself. In other words, larger lesions were found close to smaller veins and vice versa. This was also demonstrated by many noted scientists later. However, the explanation to this was that this phenomenon is directly related to the blood brain barrier breakdown.

In 1970 Charles E Lumsden also confirmed this with unmistakable images of these lesion formations near the veins. He describes that Multiple Sclerosis lesions consistently develop near the veins. He again referred to the so called Dawson fingers leading of the veins in the brain-stem. Colin W. Adams also published his result of the research into the development of cerebral Multiple Sclerosis, clearly indicated that the periventricular lesions form around the sub ependymal veins. These are the veins that are responsible for the drainage of the brain. Adams also founded that there is a close relation to the spread of Multiple Sclerosis and the course of our veins.

But with all the evidence presented above the question still remains as to what can cause this venous connection to Multiple Sclerosis. One thing that is noted is the breech of the blood brain barrier. The blood brain barrier consists of a densely packed layer of endothelial cells. The formation of the lesions close to the veins is however directly indicative of a blood brain barrier breech. This is a fact that is not disputed, as this evidence is clearly visible on a MRI enhanced scan. The blood brain barrier breach has been studied extensively in the past and the tiny holes are clearly visible under microscopic investigation. This is also the reason why Tysabri (a treatment in MS) is so effective in reducing MS Relapses, as Tysabri has the ability to reduce the blood brain barrier (BBB) breach. However what is disputed is what caused the BBB breakdown. Here is where the research is vague, with the majority being of the opinion that this is the onset of MS and the barrier breakdown is caused by an auto-immune response. A lot of studies also indicate this, but there are also a couple of studies that suggest the BBB breakdown happens as a result, or the after effect, of an immune response. Whichever way we look at it, the protective lining has tiny holes in it causing blood cells to enter the brain, thus resulting in B-Cells and killer T cells to attack the Myelin sheath over the nerve. But there is also the other side of it that certain blood cells can cross a healthy blood brain barrier by adhesion to proteins. These include Activated Leukocyte Cell Adhesion Molecule, which are induced to a pro inflammatory reaction. In other words it precedes an inflammatory reaction. It could be that this type of cell transfer can cause the onset of the immune response and in fact, this process is being investigated.

However, a recent different study suggests that a MS patient with a vascular disease can complicate MS and could explain why MS differs from person to person. Diabetes, hypertension (high blood pressure), heart disease, hyperlipidaemia (the presence of raised or abnormal levels of lipids (fatty molecules)), and peripheral (Peripheral vascular disease refers to diseases of blood vessels outside the heart and brain) disease were all included in this study. This study of co-morbidity was done on patient records only and not on clinical trials. Patients with a vascular co-morbidity seem to deteriorate more quickly and MS in these patients seems to be more aggressive.

Chronic cerebrospinal venous insufficiency (CCSVI or CCVI) is a term developed by Italian researcher Doctor Paolo Zamboni in 2008 to describe compromised blood flow in the veins draining the Central Nervous System. The theory is that our blood does not drain the way it should and there is a slow perfusion in the brain causing oxidative stress in the brain. This drainage problem is caused by a blockage in the jugular vein and Azygos vein. This is the newest and latest suggestion as to a vascular connection in Multiple Sclerosis. The researcher also theorizes that it is a congenital defect, meaning we may be born with it and that could explain why the "symptom called MS" only appears in adult years. They also suggest that by opening these blockages it could either stop or slow down MS. But the theory is in infancy, to investigate whether it causes MS still needs to be explored, as well as to what role it plays in MS. But a fact still remains that initial studies indicate that CCSVI is present in 55% of all MS patients, but it is also present in 22% of healthy controls. (Please note that I take my lead on these numbers from an official US trial and no other countries, as the numbers are different and the studies were not properly controlled).

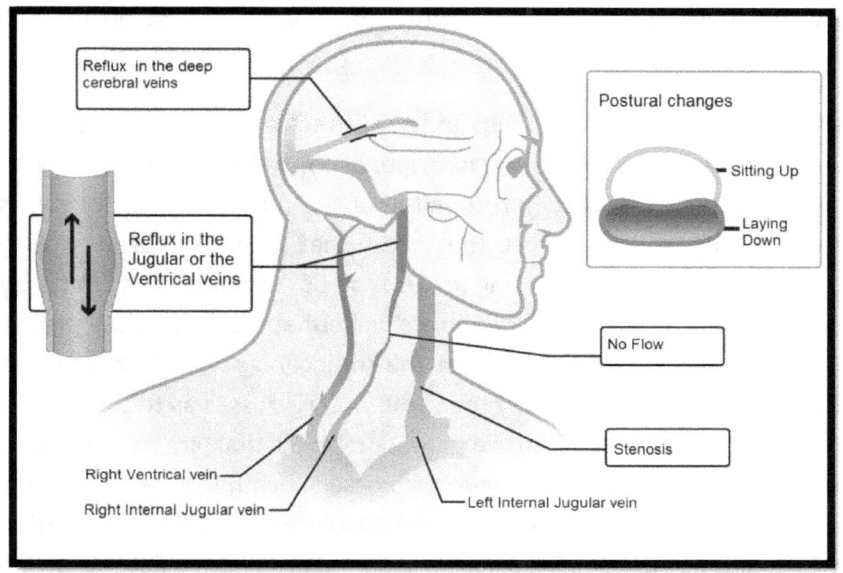

[35] CCSVI Theory (Image courtesy of Grant Groenenstein)

So let us look at what could cause CCSVI, if it is perhaps not congenital as suggested by the researcher. This seems to be highly unlikely as it does not explain the presence in healthy subjects. But what could be noted is that no two people are born with the exact same blood vessel system and it could perhaps be seen as unique as a finger print. Some persons have jugular vein valves in different positions, while others have none at all. Also noted is the fact that MS does affect people at different ages. By all logic, MS onset should then appear in a closer age range and not as varied as it is now. However looking at it as a result or complication of MS seems to make more sense. For this we need to look at the Virchow's triad, or the triangle describing what causes venous system damage. Although it is named after Virchow, it has been documented by different scientists. The triad describes three types of vascular damage. The first category, alterations in normal blood flow, refers to several situations which include turbulence, stasis, mitral stenosis, and varicose veins. The second category, injuries and/or trauma to endothelium includes damage to the veins arising from sheer stress or hypertension. The last category, alterations in the constitution of blood, has numerous possible risk factors such as hyper viscosity, deficiency of ant thrombin, nephritic syndrome, changes after severe trauma or burn, disseminated cancer, late pregnancy and delivery, race, age, whether the patient is a smoker, and obesity.

Looking at the above triad, we need to look at the second category applying to MS being damage to vessels being endothelial damage, or for better words damage to the blood brain barrier. One aspect that is noted is the mention of sheer stress causing this type of damage. This is also the theory that CCSVI is caused by long term sheer stress. However, what is lacking in this type of theory is that CCSVI is on the vein side; hence the likelihood of sheer stress will not apply here as the jugular and Azygos veins transport blood back from the brain and spinal cord and are mostly free flowing and not influenced by the same sheer stresses as to the arterial side. However, oxidative stress due to oxygen-poor blood that are trapped in a stasis or turbulence in the jugular as a result of blockages could cause this effect, but again it is more likely that it will not take years to present itself. An indication of this is the Putman studies on dogs and the damage due to oxidative stress happens in a very short time span. The longest test on a dog in the Putman study was 12 months.

What seems to be more likely is the stenosis of the vein is a direct result of endothelial damage as a result of a MS immune response. Endothelial damage is, in most cases, a predecessor of stenosis or thrombosis in veins. In other words, the stenosis as described in CCSVI, can be as a blockage caused by scar tissue build-up on the blood vessel lining or valves as a result of endothelial damage. The fact that scar tissue in the vein was found in tested samples of blood vessels in CCSVI indicates that endothelial cell damage is rather a predecessor of the stenosis. Still this does not explain the 22% of healthy controls that present with CCSVI. But many other diseases could explain this phenomenon as not all endothelial cell damages results in a breach of the blood brain barrier. The endothelial cells can be damaged by other inflammatory diseases as well, without a breach of the blood brain barrier. One big culprit here could be Epstein Bar Virus. EBV does cause endothelial damage, and 95% of all adults are exposed to EBV in their life. Smoking can also damage the endothelial layer. One aspect that can be a result of a congenital defects are incorrect valves in the veins but these are limited cases, and there are also other noted stenosis in these patients and not the valves alone. What is lacking in the CCSVI theory is the explanation as to why the blood brain barrier breaks down. The stasis, turbulence or even the shear stress that may be indicated in CCSVI still does not fully explain the blood brain barrier breakdown. The researchers speculate that this is due to sheer or oxidative stress, but does not clearly indicate the process.

But these blockages could in respect certainly affect the disease prognosis and recovery, as with an added drainage factor of oxygen poor blood away from the damage blood brain barrier, could significantly decrease the repair process. Thus this is certainly an added avenue to research. Reflux oxygen poor blood into a brain with an added factor such as a blood brain barrier breach can certainly not be good for the disease nor the brain itself. But the cause and effect of CCSVI needs to be clearly researched to determine this link and to see what possible roll it could play in our recovery. But it still leaves one very big unanswered question as to why this is present in only 55% of MS patients and in 22% of healthy controls. Of interest will be to follow the healthy controls to see if they develop MS and when.

**Dual receptor killer cells in Multiple Sclerosis**, could it a possible be a cause of Multiple Sclerosis? The University of Washington Department of Immunology scientists have conducted the study, which was published in June 2010, in Nature Immunology. The result of this study suggests that MS may be caused by a dual receptor in certain peoples CD+8 cells.

The researcher set out to genetically engineer mice to overproduce CD+8 killer white blood cells. These are the white blood cells that have the ability to cross the blood brain barrier. The blood brain barrier protects the brain from blood cells entering the brain. The normal function of these killer white blood cells is to protect the body from a viral attack of tumor cells. The researchers then went ahead and introduced a Myelin basic protein virus in these mice. The reaction they were hoping for was that the virus will activate the response from the CD+8 and in a sense, commission the troops to fight the Myelin basic protein virus and set off a cascade of events that will eventually cause an out of control reaction.

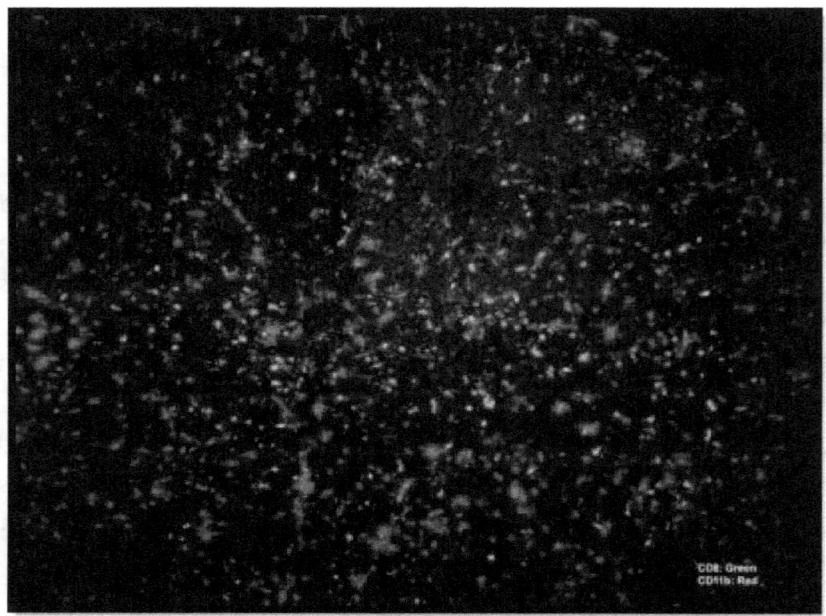

[36] "A section of brain from a mouse with multiple sclerosis-like disease induced by viral infection. The fluorescently stained image shows a type of killer white blood cell, called CD8+ T cells (colored green), invading the brain and attracting other immune cells (red) that degrade the nerve protein Myelin." (Image courtesy of Joan Goverman lab at the University of Washington)

Exactly this happened, the response caused the over production of killer cells and when the Myelin basic virus was destroyed, the killer cells went on to attack the Myelin in the central nervous system. And true to form, these mice developed a Multiple Sclerosis like disease. This is probably the closest match of animal induced Multiple Sclerosis model. It ties in with research that MS develops as an overreaction of the Immune system following perhaps a viral agent like Epstein Bar Virus which closely resembles Myelin protein.

But to their surprise, some of the mice that were not exposed to the Myelin basic protein virus started to develop a MS like disease as well. When they carried on cross breeding these genetically engineered mice they notice some dual receptor CD+8 cells. In the human CD+8 cells in normally co-receptor cells, in other words, it has only one receptor or molecule binding to it. Effectively the CD+8 with dual receptors recognised the Myelin basic protein virus as well as Myelin as a foreign invader and went on to attack the Myelin over the nerves, even when not exposed to the Myelin basic protein virus. These dual receptor cells crossed the blood brain barrier and attached itself to Myelin, starting an immune reaction that commanded more killer cells and helper cells to attack the Myelin on the central nervous system.

What it effectively means is that normal people produce CD+8 cells in the course of everyday existence, but that some of these killer cells maybe predisposed to develop dual receptors. We already know that persons with Multiple Sclerosis do overproduce CD+8 as this was proven in studies in the past. This is one of the reason they suspect a viral attack causing a cascade of events commanding more killer cells to fight a viral infection with a protein similar to Myelin, but then goes on to attack Myelin itself. The fact that these dual receptors were found could indicate that in the case of an over production of killer cells, the dual receptor CD+8 resulting as a direct cause of overproduction of these cells could attack to Myelin itself by attaching the Myelin and setting of the cascade of events that leads to an MS attack. This opens a new avenue to research to test humans for these dual receptors as well.

This could explain that a genetic factor to produce these dual receptors in certain individuals could lead to Multiple Sclerosis, while certain people who produce co-receptor cells may not develop Multiple Sclerosis. This research could possible lead to the cause and effect of Multiple Sclerosis.

**Acrolein may cause of Multiple Sclerosis.**

A recent finding suggests that Acrolein may be involved in the cause of Multiple Sclerosis.

Safe human consumption of Acrolein is 2 parts per millilitre. This is a very small dosage. Acrolein was used as a chemical weapon in World War two, but it was never classified as a chemical weapon, by the chemical weapons act. The effects of Acrolein were studied before on lab rats and have shown an increase in Cancer tumour forming cells when consumed, but not inhaled. In 2006 studies have shown that Acrolein produced by cigarette smoke may lead to the increase of lung cancer.

This study is the first investigate the direct effects of Acrolein in the human nervous system. Acrolein is also a by-product produced in the body after nerve cell damage. Nerve cell deaths may be counteracted by the administration of Hydralazine (Apresoline), a smooth muscle relaxant and a treatment for high blood pressure. Studies on this are on-going, and Hydralazine prevented nerve cell death, after the consumption of Acrolein in mice. This on-going study suggests that Multiple Sclerosis may be slowed down by Hydralazine. In this study of MS mice, elevated Acrolein levels were cut in half, by the introduction of Hydralazine. If this is the case, treating Multiple Sclerosis with Hydralazine, may reduce the degree of progression.

Acrolein consumption and inhalation leads to lung infections and irritation. Acrolein is used in Chemotherapy, but is counteracted by expectorants. Acrolein is used in the preparation of polyester resin, polyurethane, propylene glycol, acrylic acid, and glycerol. It is also used as a contact herbicide to control submersed and floating weeds, as well as algae, in irrigation canals. It is also a by-product found in wastewater treatment. The environmental protection agency has strict regulation as to the allowable parts of Acrolein in wastewater.

This is one of the most common products used globally and is also found in one of the biggest pollutant, namely auto mobile exhaust. It is a by-product of cigarette smoke. It is used in the preparation of propylene glycol. Propylene glycol is a very common product used in a wide variety of products. Glycol is used as in the coolant system in cars. It is also found in saline solutions in medicine. Your standard freezer jacket and ice packs contains glycol as well. Glycol is very toxic, and a couple of cases of deliberate glycol poising were reported in USA, leading to death. One teaspoon of Glycol over ten days will kill you.

This study is still on-going and there are plans afoot to introduce anti-acrolein trials in Multiple Sclerosis. Purdue University researchers are planning a trial of an already approved drug Hydralazine, for use in Multiple Sclerosis treatment. Yet again an old favourite, oxidative stress is revisited in Multiple Sclerosis. Time will tell if this research leads to anything conclusive.

# Treating my first Multiple Sclerosis relapse.

Back in 1993, the only treatment for Multiple Sclerosis was Steroids for a relapse and is still the case today. All other drugs were still experimental and new to the market. My first introduction to this treatment followed the afternoon of the last test.

Intravenous corticosteroid (Steroids) treatment consists of 1000mg of Solu-Medrol daily for five days. The main aim of this treatment is to slow down the immune response, or the attack that your body is mounting on your nervous system, and stripping the Myelin off your Nerve Acton. Corticosteroids are used to supress your own immune system, slowing down the attack of killer cells in your blood. This treatment is normally given in the hospital either as an in-house treatment or as an outpatient. Today; Doctors tend to limit this treatment to 3 days.

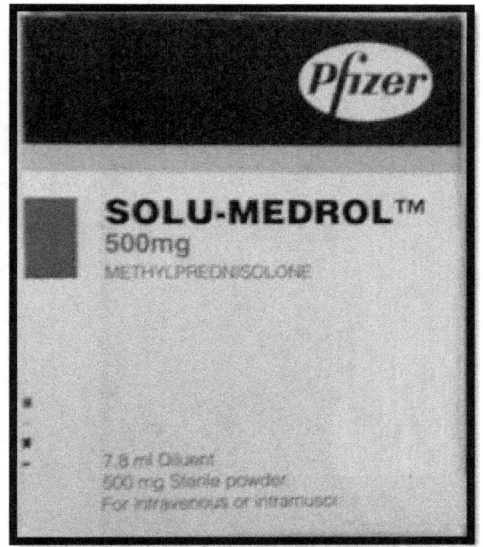

[37] Solu-Medrol (Image from one of my treatments)

The high dose Solu-Medrol is infused over a period of normally three hours. As an outpatient, the treatment time can be reduced but care must be taken that the infusion is not too fast. When your face starts to feel hot or your vein or arm develops a burning sensation, rather ask the nurses to slow down the process a bit.

The human body tolerates the treatment quite well, and the side effects are little and manageable.

Common side effects include increased appetite, increased energy and irritability, insomnia and upset stomach. Rare but serious side effects include psychosis, stomach ulcers, aseptic bone necrosis, infections, irregular heart rhythms and blood clots. Solu-Medrol must be given with caution in patients with hypertension, diabetes or a history of stomach ulcers, so please advise your doctor if you do suffer from these. It also has no harmful effect after the first trimester of pregnancy.

You will also experience water retention to an extent, which will leave you looking bloated, like a blow fish for a couple of days after the treatment. It leaves a very metallic aftertaste in your mouth. I dealt with this by eating some sweets during and after the treatment.

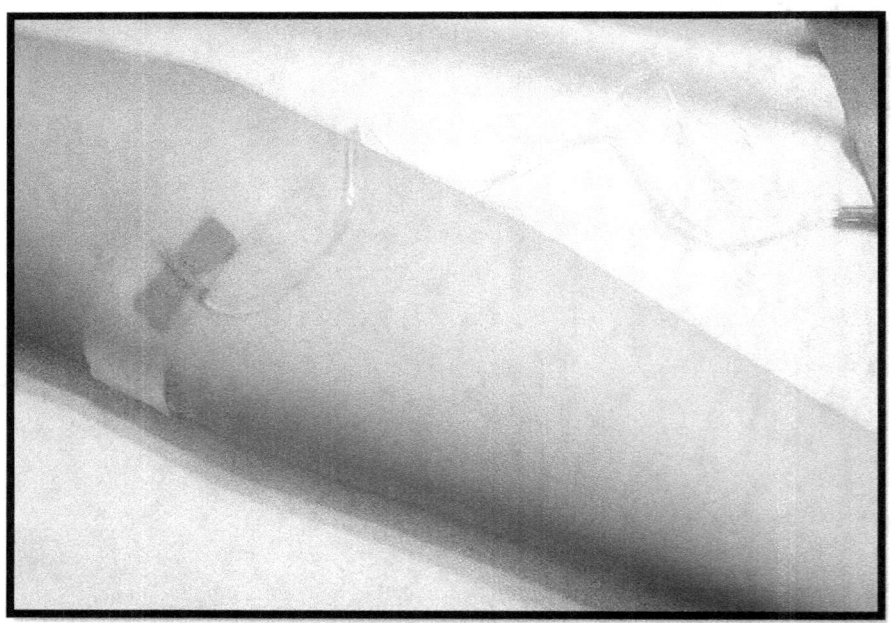

[38] Intravenous Corticosteroid Treatment (Image source: Wikipedia. Author: Wilfredo Rodriguez)

After the treatment course you will be given a tapered down dosage of Corticosteroid in a pill form. The tapered down dosage varies from patient to patient. It is an oral dosage, not as high as the Intravenous dosage, usually around 100mg per day; reduced by 10mg every second day, but some doctors reduce it every day. This taper down dosage is given to reduce the risk of an Addison Crisis. This can happen as a direct result of the high dose Corticosteroid. In a Addison Crisis, the body's adrenal glands do not produce sufficient steroid hormones; as a result of the high dose steroids received the days before and the brain is sending a message that the body has enough steroids, therefor do not produce more. Signs of this are fatigue, light headedness upon standing or while upright, muscle weakness, fever, weight loss, difficulty in standing up, anxiety, nausea, vomiting, diarrhoea, headache, sweating, changes in mood and personality, and joint and muscle pains. This is not common in all patients, but in a small percentage this is a reality.  And as the old saying, goes prevention is better than cure.

Continued use of high does cortisone can lead to osteoporosis or brittle bones, and schizophrenia. In the early days of cortisone treatment, schizophrenia was noted, and the treatments were therefore given only on a necessary basis.

Patients must take great care after a cortisone treatment for secondary opportunistic infections. Remember your body's immune system is now suppressed and picking up the common flu can lead to severe lung infections. The most common of this is Fungal Pneumonia. Your immune system is now suppressed and the chances of picking up an airborne fungal spore are high. It is however treatable and you need to inform your doctor if you have received any cortisone treatments in the weeks leading up to the Pneumonia to rule out the chances of him treating the wrong type of Pneumonia.

Other opportunistic infections are real too and rather have any unusual symptoms checked out by the doctor before they get worse, or you may need more aggressive treatment.

This was my introduction to my first course of steroid treatment in my life, and I must say not a pleasant one. I have a term for it "Gummy Berry Juice". I coined the expression after realising that eating Gummy Berry sweets helps the awful metallic taste in your mouth. I am adding a final word of warning to all that receive this treatment. Always be in close proximity of the toilet, for as the water retention starts to dissipate, you are definitely going to need to go more often than usual, to find the necessary relief or to put it bluntly, peeing is going to be one of your favourite past times during the days that follow.

After my first treatment I was allowed to go home from hospital for a couple of days. As for my eyesight and numbness, there was a bit of relief but not as much as I have hoped for. Spending nine days in Hospital can be quite stressful, and missing the comforts of home was getting a bit depressing. This was not a permanent "get free out of jail card", and I had to be back in seven days to determine whether the treatment had benefited me or not. I could now at least distinguish larger objects in front of me but as far as reading, watching television and all those other joys in life that healthy sighted people take for granted, were not yet destined for me.

A week later after some much relief from the dreaded hospital food, I found myself back in the neurologist's office on the Monday morning. Another series of test followed, not as complicated as the first round, consisting only on normal reflex tests. As far as my eyesight was concerned, the big chief was a bit concerned. He cautioned me that there was not a great improvement in my ability to see, and suggested that we do another steroid course. I was a bit reluctant to go through another treatment, and the chief also expressed his concern. But after a dialogue we decided that in order to save my eyesight it was a risk worth taking.

There I was back in Hospital for another couple of days, ready but not quite willing for the next rounds of steroids. Another Visual Evoke Potential test was done late in the morning. My only guess was that although there are certain indicators that a normal neurological eye exam can pick up, they need to make absolutely sure that I am on the level with them. The VEP confirmed the suspicion of optical nerve involvement. I was armed for the side effect, the metallic taste in my mouth and brought a week's supply of "Gummy Berry Sweets" along, expecting this would happen.

Another five days of Gummy Berry juice started, and the awful tasting hospital food was my immediate future. Accepting this gracefully I set of to the hospital ward again. Hooked up on an IV line and dragging this metal tripod around wherever I went, especially for the nicotine fixes, was now an all too familiar part of my day. This visit was however, different. After the third day my eyesight was slowly getting better and with about 60% of the sight in my left eye and the numbness subsiding, I was certain that I was back to my old normal self.

I completed my steroid course and spent the rest of the weekend in hospital, anxiously awaiting Monday. The day came and finally the neurologist sat down and talked to me. He told me given my past history and the past three weeks he can definitely say that I have Multiple Sclerosis. How severe; he could not say, and what will eventually happen to me is still uncertain. He did mention that the disease varies from person to person, and if I am lucky I would be able to live a normal life for the next 10-15 years. Worst case was my eyesight, and given the problems I had with my right eye, I might lose my sight in a very short period of time or I could end up in a wheel chair in five years. I admired this man for his honesty, but a feeling of anger built up towards him when told there was no cure. Also given the loss of my vision he was going to put me on medical disability. This was the last piece of information I actually wanted to hear, I was not yet thirty, and essentially my life was over, or so I thought.

The rest of that year, I had two relapses requiring steroid treatment. The constant reminder was ever present in my daily life with some blurred vision from day to day, and the about 80% sight I had in one eye only. I had lost my job and was battling to make ends meet.  Was it not for an insurance policy pay-out, I probably would have lost everything in life.

I will go into more detail about drug treatments and preventative medication in Multiple Sclerosis in a later chapter in this book.

# Being Diagnosed with Multiple Sclerosis, what now?

You have just walked out of hospital or seen the neurologist and been given the diagnosis that you have Multiple Sclerosis, so what happens next?

This is when you need to make some very big decisions and some very important lifestyle changes. Most of us lose control at this stage, but I am going to try and give you choices. These choices could enable you to make informed decisions. There are a couple of ways to make this all the more bearable for yourself, and could also help you in your life ahead. Note that I say "your life ahead", as this is not the end of your life but the beginning of a new chapter in your life. What you do from now on will determine the rest of your life. You are likely to go through the certain stages of emotional feelings and thoughts that most of us go through after our diagnosis.

The first of these stages is denial and it happens to all of us, and certainly after the recovery of your first relapse. You are now over your relapse and you feel fine and you are likely to feel normal again. "I feel fine, the Doctors could be wrong I don't have MS". For about 5% of patients this is certainly true, but a good neurologist will not wrongfully diagnose you after meeting some of the criteria for Multiple Sclerosis that have been ascertained by these tests. In certain patients you do get what is known as Clinical Isolated Syndrome, in other words, you only have one attack in your entire life and the symptoms disappear for ever. This diagnosis will only be given if you do not meet all the criteria of Multiple Sclerosis and most cases you do not present with a second attack. In 95% of all cases, the diagnosis of Multiple Sclerosis is definite and no matter how you try to deny it, you still have Multiple Sclerosis. The first thing you should do is not to dwell on this point too long; because the sooner you accept you have Multiple Sclerosis, the better it will be for you.

The next step is to get all the info available on Multiple Sclerosis out there. Do be careful in the selection of reading material on the subject. I did it the old fashion way, by going to libraries and read all I could about the disease. The internet is probably, in my opinion, the worst place to get first time information on Multiple

Sclerosis. There are so many false promises and hopes being published on it, unless you could get it from a recognised organisation. The best place to get this information is at the local chapter of a Multiple Sclerosis society. They have been around for many years and have a credible amount of information on Multiple Sclerosis. If there is not a chapter or MS organisation near you, write to one. They will be more than willing to send you the information. Read through all this material and digest it all. This info will guide you through the rest of your life. Once you have informed yourself on the basic facts on multiple sclerosis, it should be safe to get onto the internet. Join a support page and meet some friends on it. But, be very careful of opportunists. Multiple Sclerosis is a disease that is fear driven, and many fall into the trap of trying to find a miracle cure out there. 99% of these operators have one thing in common, and that is to get you into their trap and use their powers of persuasion to follow their so-called cures. Guide yourself with the Societies' recognised information, and for the better part avoid all the so called "cures". Do not let yourself be fooled into believing all that is on the internet. We live in an era with very modern and fast spreading information, and this is called the World Wide Web. It has it positive side, but it also has a very negative side to it. Avoid the pitfalls on the internet as this will lead you to false hope in most cases.

Now that you are informed you have to decide; do I tell my family, friends and co-workers? This is a definite yes, because the support of these friend and colleagues will help you a great deal in your future life. Or in certain cases; the lack of support will also determine what you do in your life. The information that you have armed yourself with now comes in handy. Use this information and pamphlets as a tool to educate others in your life. Spread the information to the important people in your life and rally them behind you. But do it in a constructive way, so that they don't pity you as this is not what you need. You need to surround yourself with positive people and friends. You are not over the wall yet, and the more positive backing you receive, the better it is for you. But they also need to understand what to expect regarding your physical abilities. This education is an on-going process, because as your Multiple Sclerosis changes so will your physical abilities and certainly while you are in relapse, you may require the help and understanding of these people in your life. But this is also the point where you should not be stubborn. Accept the help that is given to you. It will go a long way in your recovery process.

Now comes the important part; do not give up hope. There is a good Latin saying "Dum spiro, spero, "While I breath, I hope"". This is not the stage to crawl in a corner and give up. Giving up is the worst thing that you can do now. It is understandable to feel helpless while you have a relapse, but as soon as this relapse is over, get back out there and live life again. Set goals for yourself to achieve, but know your limitations. Do not set impossible goals to achieve. Get constructive, get involved. If you do still work, try to remain there as long as possible, but also do not over exert yourself or put too much stress on yourself. Avoid stress whenever possible, as this is one of the worst enemies of Multiple Sclerosis. If you are not working, get involved with volunteer work, but occupy your mind and keep busy with something else. This will go a long way in helping you. The important part is to remain active for as long as possible.  Take up a hobby, do something that interests you and keeps you from falling into a state of depression. Remember a healthy mind supports a healthy body. Stay positive as positive thoughts will lead to a positive life.

Change your lifestyle; this is very important. Forget about the past, the future is now and that is what counts. Change your diet, follow a healthy eating plan. But going healthy does not mean to go to the extreme e.g. vegetarian. You do not need to make drastic changes, but avoid fatty food, and eat more of the so called "heart healthy" foods. Eat a normal balanced diet. But it does not mean you cannot reward yourself with some treats every now and then. You are still you and there is no need to stop eating out and socialising. But the key is moderation. A big question that is likely on everyone's mind is do I stop having alcohol? Again moderation applies here as well. Have a glass of wine or a drink or two, but be conservative.

In comes the next step; exercise. This is a very complicated issue as you can only do what your body allows you too. Avoid exercise that will raise your core temperature. Exercise in moderation, for the longer your muscle stays active the longer you will be active. A very important part is to get back into action after a relapse. The better your muscles are trained the better your ability will be to handle Multiple Sclerosis. I am not saying getting trained to run the New York marathon. There are exercises like yoga that can get you in just as good shape without exerting yourself. Yoga type exercise will keep your muscle toned and supple, and this helps a lot to avoid muscle wasting away and going into spasm. For those who can afford it, get physical therapy. But the important part is train your body to deal with Multiple Sclerosis. If you can do small exercises while you are sitting and watching TV etc., if you have legs that spasm, stretch and do subtle exercise. Put a tennis ball under your foot and roll it, this will even help for foot drop.

Listen to your body; it has a story to tell. Look for early warning signs of a flare up or relapse. Know the early signs like numbness, painful eyes, facial pains etc. When you see the warning signs, get treatment rather sooner than later. Your primary physician or neurologist is trained to look for other early warning signs. Go to them if you see a sign of a possible attack. The sooner you get treated the quicker you will recover. Avoid opportunistic infections like flu or any viral infection. Don't let this go untreated as it could trigger an immune response. Avoid contact with sick people if possible. For those mothers of young children, this is going to be extremely difficult. The motherly instinct will take over, and I think it is unavoidable as your child takes priority. Get vaccinated every year for flu and do so for your whole family, but check that the vaccine is safe to use in Multiple Sclerosis. Rest when your body tells you too. This is very important in Multiple Sclerosis.

Inform yourself as to the treatments available, as disease modifying drugs (DMD) can go a long way to help slow down your Multiple Sclerosis. For those that can't afford it, find out from your local MS Chapter or neurologist as to drug sponsored help programmes. Certain countries do have them. Get the right DMD, if the one does not work inform your neurologist as there are other options. It is likely that your neurologist will not put you on a DMD before your second attack. This is just good practice and do not worry about it then. Always inform your primary if you are on DMD as certain medicine does not react well in combination with DMD's. Also now keep a diary of all new and strange symptoms as this will come in handy in the future. Take this to the Doctor with each visit and keep it up to date. This is the most important part of your literature for the future. It is your MS Biography, keep it up to date. It is now part of the rest of your life. Lastly listen to the doctors as to what you can and cannot do.

Now comes my last part of important information. Having Multiple Sclerosis does not mean you should stop living; follow all the important guidelines and you can live a long productive life albeit with a bit more difficulty. Never give up hope, there are important medical advances made in the field of Multiple Sclerosis, and in the near future, the new line of treatments and medicine will go a long way to help our battle against Multiple Sclerosis.

# My personal experience with the devastating symptoms of Multiple Sclerosis

My personal experience with Multiple Sclerosis started in my teens, and with what doctors then dismissed as growing pains, etc. but I can almost with certainty say these were my first symptoms. Between the ages of 13-15 years, I often experienced a sort of numbness with terrible pains in my legs. To describe the feeling I had in my legs would be like comparing it to an elastic band wrapped around your finger until it goes numb and develops pins and needles. This sensation is called Paresthesia. It normally starts with just pins and needles and later spread to numbness of the limb. I still recall my mother saying that I probably sat on my leg and it had fallen asleep. Today I experience these feelings on a regular basis, and I can positively identify this as my first symptom. Paresthesia includes symptoms such as numbness, pins and needles, burning sensation, itching and tingling or vibrating sensations.

Paresthesia is normally one of the first signs of a pending Multiple Sclerosis relapse. The severity of Paresthesia also differs from mild to very extreme. Your motor skills may be impaired and especially your fine motor skills. A simple task like picking up a pencil can become a bit daunting. Sensory Ataxia is in most cases also present. This is lack of co-ordination and position sensing, making small tasks into huge tasks.

Environmental factors play a huge role in Paresthesia, with heat being the most common one. This is in medical terms referred to as pseudo exacerbation. MS patients tend not to do well in heat. Any temperature above the average cool range can affect us very badly. The hotter it gets the worst the Paresthesia gets. Temporary relief from heat can be found in a good air conditioned home, keeping the temperature around 22⁰ Celsius or 72⁰ Fahrenheit. Simple cooler vests can also be worn to lower the body core temperature.

Another major factor influencing MS Symptoms and Paresthesia is fatigue. The more tired we get the worst the symptoms get. However Multiple Sclerosis does cause fatigue as well. Avoid being overtired as it will just worsen your situation. Rest as much as possible, the less tired the body is the, more of a chance the relapse will go over quicker.   Paresthesia tends to be worse at night and can interfere with your sleep.

Paresthesia will go away after most relapses and treatments, but a small reminder of it usually remains long after treatment and may, remain depending on the type of Multiple Sclerosis you have.

The second symptom is one that I had to deal with for most of my teenage years. Proprioceptive Dysfunction is the feeling of being clumsy and causing the patient to trip or fall. This also leads to certain dysfunction in picking up or placing an object. Most patients in the onset of MS see these symptoms as being clumsy, and not due to MS therefore they don't seek medical advice. It is only when these symptoms disrupts their daily life that they seek help. In my teenage years I was always clumsy, and still am today, although it is much worse than then. I was always the kid with no ball sense. So for me, running was a better option. In another life I would probably have played ball sports, but the couple of times I did partake, the outcome was not the best. I have tripped on many an occasion in my life, but the worst one I could remember was tripping on a horse bridge a couple of years ago, landing head first in the river.

The third symptom in my early years was probably the most distinguished marker of Multiple Sclerosis in my life.

When I was about 13 years old I had the misfortune of injuring my right eye with a catapult after a childhood prank that went wrong. We were living in a small town with only one doctor. After the accident the Doctor was called to my house to examine the severity of the injury. Growing up, my parents were not wealthy, and we could not take his advice to see an Ophthalmologist. A couple of phone calls later, it was decided that I had to spend the next week flat on my back in bed. The outcome at the end was not very good and I developed a cataract in the lens. I could still see but my vision was blurred and with a sort of a white haze over it.

During my senior years of high school, and especially at age 16, I was sent home on many occasions with hay fever. But this was not a typical hay fever in my opinion. Reflecting back today, the onset would start suddenly in the morning and especially on hot days. It only affected my right eye for some strange reason. On the occasion that I went to see a doctor about it, he diagnosed it as hay fever and I was placed on anti-histamines. My right eye would get totally pink with blood and the white appeared swollen, compared to the lens. There were definite indicators of some form of swelling of the blood vessels in the eye.

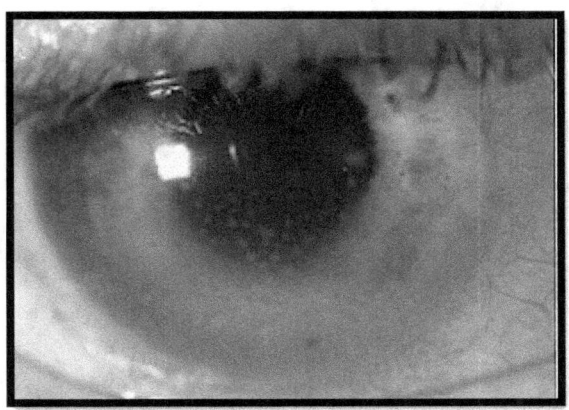

[39] Uveitis (Image courtesy of anonymous patient)

Uveitis and Phlebitis are normally concurrent and I am dealing with this symptom in my next chapter. Looking back today, this was probably my first major indicator that I have had Symptoms of Multiple Sclerosis since as early as the age of 13.

At the age twenty I eventually went to see an Ophthalmologist, and his suggestion was to remove the optic lens in the right eye and fit me with contact lenses. I have a big pain tolerance, but let me tell you removing an eye lens in those years was an extremely painful operation. There was not a variety of smart drugs, and this was done under general anaesthesia. A couple of weeks later, I was given a contact lens to wear, and had again nearly perfect 20/20 vision. In 1988 I went for another operation to get a permanent lens implant. The eye doctor doing the operation was a bit sceptical as my optic disc was pale. The optic disc is the disc where the retina meets the eye nerve. Enquiring about my vision, I told him that my sight is blurry sometimes. He noted it, but still did the transplant.

Little did I know the value of that pale disc and what was it meant. A year after the lens implant I started getting blurred vision at times, but with a difference. It was painful as well. I went to my general practitioner, and he was puzzled. Giving me a bit of pain relief, I was sent packing back to the Ophthalmologist. He described it as possible Optic Neuritis.

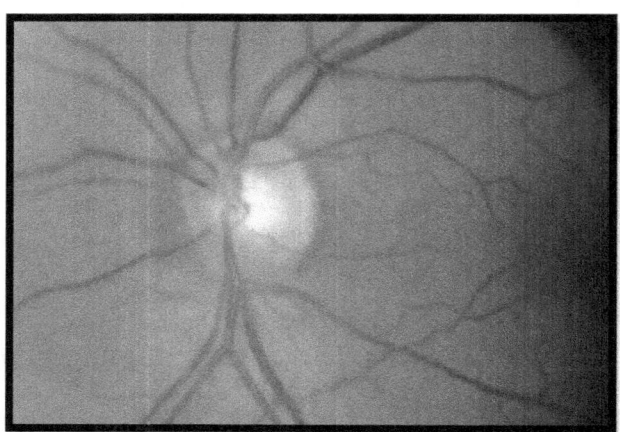

[40] Optic Neuritis (Image source: National Library of Medicine (NLM))

The picture clearly depicts Optic Neuritis with the retina meeting the optic disc. In this the pale optic disc can be clearly seen whereas in a healthy disc it would appear to be pink. Optic Neuritis can be mild to very painful especially with eye movements. The most common cause of Optic Neuritis is Multiple Sclerosis and about 50% of all Multiple Sclerosis patients will develop Optic Neuritis in their life. There are a few other causes of Optic Neuritis like Lyme disease, Herpes Zoster and Diabetes. Having Optic Neuritis only without any other neurological symptoms does not mean that you have Multiple Sclerosis. In the early 1980- 90 the link between Optic Neuritis and Multiple Sclerosis was not highly emphasized, but the picture has changed since then. Ophthalmologists do tend to look at Optic Neuritis more closely today and are on the lookout for possible immune disorders' involvement as well. In a human being, the optic nerve is the only direct extension of the brain, and the only part that can be examined non-intrusively.

The symptoms of Optic Neuritis are painful eyes, with the sudden onset of vision loss. The vision loss appears normally within 24-48 hours of the first symptoms appearing. The first symptoms are sudden blurred or "foggy" vision, reduced light perception, and certain amounts of colour loss and flashes of lights when the eyes are moved. Most do not notice the colour loss, but red is the first colour to disappear from the spectrum.

I did not have any other markers of Multiple Sclerosis then and was only treated for Optic Neuritis. I did receive a couple of injections behind the eye socket with what I today perceive as a corticosteroid injection. I had at that stage in my life suffered, from severe Optic Neuritis, and was on heavy pain medication. My sight in my right side was about 5%. Together with the Ophthalmologist, the decision was taken to rather numb the optic nerve where it exits the brain. A Retrobulbar alcohol injection was done behind the eyes. Knowing full well that I may never fully recover my eyesight in that eye, I opted rather for pain free days since it has been now about four months of living with Optic Neuritis.

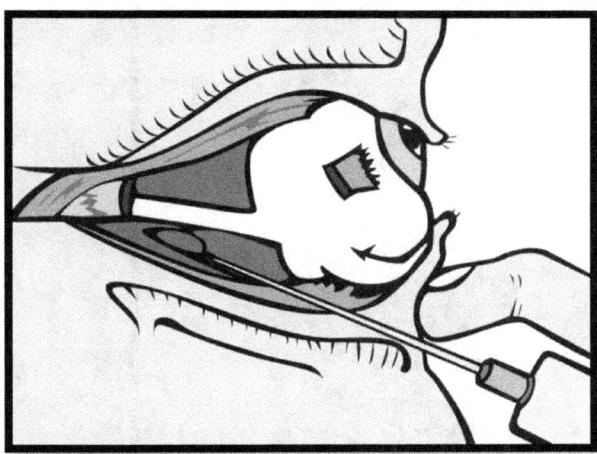

[41] Retrobulbar Alcohol Block (Image courtesy of Grant Groenenstein)

Today, this is my most common symptom, but also my watch dog symptom. At the slightest hint of an Optic Neuritis attack, I hop off to the clever people for a closer look. This is my early alarm, and it has not let me down yet. This symptom was the one that lead to my diagnosis.

Two years passed with no new problems until one day after a visit to the dentist. The visit went off quite well, but what followed was a nightmare. I met a new symptom a couple of days later, long after the pain of extracting the tooth had disappeared. Suddenly it felt as if someone was pushing a red hot iron to the right lower side of my face and jaw, with jolting electric shock pain.

Facial Trigeminal Neuralgia is also a symptom of Multiple Sclerosis resulting in a painful sensation of the facial area. The three trigeminal nerves in the face are normally affected in the facial area. Certain criteria of Trigeminal neuralgia are so severe that it can make it difficult to speak or eat without suffering severe pain in the side of the face.

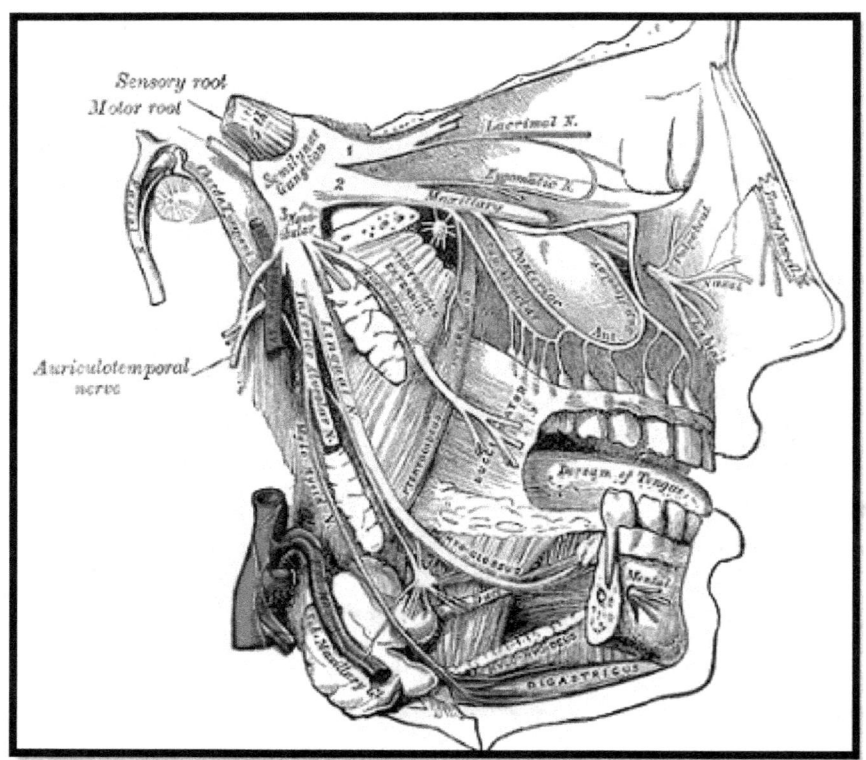

[42] Trigeminal Nerves (Image source: Wikipedia)

Trigeminal Neuralgia (TN) is probably the worst symptom of pain a Multiple Sclerosis patient could suffer in his life it is no wonder it was called the Suicide Disease. In the early days of medicine around the 18th century, many of those who suffered from this rather opted for suicide than living with this pain.

Trigeminal Neuralgia is caused by cranial nerves being affected by Multiple Sclerosis but is also found in other patients without MS as well. The cause in

Multiple Sclerosis is the demyelination and lesions on the cranial nerves and in other cases normally caused by compression of the nerves. The Cranial nerves exits the brain below the frontal cortex, and splits into different routes. The lower half of the jaw and side of the face nerve are mostly affected. The middle and lower branch of the Trigeminal nerve are normally affected. Nearly 1 in 20,000 people suffer from TN, but in MS it is fairly rare, with only about 4% afflicted by it.

The symptoms are an intense sharp pain feeling like an electric jolt. The pain is mostly short lived lasting from a few seconds to a couple of minutes. Attacks usually affect one side of the face at a time, lasting from several seconds to a few minutes and repeats up to hundreds of times a day. TN can extend as far back as the ear, and easily mistaken as an ear ache or tooth pain. The bouts of attacks can last for weeks on end with no relief.

Trigeminal neuralgia is triggered by chewing, drinking or brushing your teeth. Loud noises can also trigger it but this is rarely reported. The pain is so intense, and in some cases it can require hospitalization and intravenous painkillers. In very few cases surgery is required to cut the affected trigeminal nerve leaving the person paralyzed in that side of the face, however this is very rarely done. Treatment consists mostly of painkillers and in some cases doing a mandibular local anaesthetic block, or in plain English, an injection of anaesthetics at the root where the cranial nerve exits the brain. I had one of these done and experienced some temporary relief. Other medication to treat this consists mostly of strong painkillers or anti-epileptic drugs.

In my case I had a tooth extracted, and till today I am not quite sure whether the pain in the teeth was actually toothache or the onset of Trigeminal neuralgia. TN is also considered an early indicator of Multiple Sclerosis.

A last but very troublesome symptom for me was the Multiple Sclerosis "HUG". There is still not a lot of medical information of this particular sign in MS, but many a patient will tell you that they do experience it.

I had short episodes of panic attacks for unexplained reasons and a feeling that I could not breathe. The attacks were short lived and latest about two hours or so, and cost me a couple of visits to the emergency department at the hospital. It was not prescribed to anything. Later my problems started getting worse. In 1989, I started developing severe panic attacks with chest pain and was sent to hospital for some tests, including blood sugar level and all that could cause this. Nothing seemed to help and these attacks seem to get worse over time. I was sent to a psychologist and received electro shock therapy (won't recommend this for any one, it is utter hell). No specific diagnosis was done at that stage. And as suddenly as this came, it disappeared.

Four months before my diagnoses I started having these panic attacks again and was hyperventilating without any reason and had severe chest pains. The doctor was of the opinion that it was rather again a mental factor and this landed me up at psychologist yet again. I was put on an anti-depressant and this seemed to help. There were no mental issues that caused these attacks. The reason way I say there were no mental issues to cause this, might be due to the fact that I was very "happy go-lucky" all my life. At the age of 48 I am still sort of the same, nothing in this world can make me feel down. Eventually this also disappeared with time and I was on my way to complete health again. Only after being diagnosed and reading up on Multiple Sclerosis I figured out it was a MS Hug.

**The MS Hug** is caused by a lesion in the spinal cord and is classified as a neuropathic pain. Basically what happens is the small muscle between the ribs called the intercostal muscle, tends to spasm. At times the diaphragm muscle also spasms. The feeling it causes differs from patient to patient. To describe it best; most of the patients that experience this will tell you that they need space for their lungs to breath. It feels like your torso is wrapped in a pressure bandage. To some, it may be a mild pain but it can be so severe for some people that it feels like a crushing pain. Some will tell you that they feel like they are having a heart attack. Patient say they feel like they can't breathe or it is painful when breathing. About 45% of MS patients experience this feeling although this figure has never been acknowledged. It can last for a couple of seconds or as long as a couple of hours. It is exacerbated when the patient is fatigued or stressed. Neurologists or doctors tend to attribute this to panic attacks or stress.

The above symptoms are what I experienced before I got my official diagnoses. It was a long hard road getting there, but it was a relief to finally know what was wrong with me. Presenting with a variety of symptoms, that doctors cannot actually pinpoint a diagnosis is frustrating. I have first-hand knowledge of what many of my fellow MS patient continue to experience on a daily basis. One thing is for certain, and I may step on some Doctors toes here, when you consult with them presenting with a painful condition and no direct course is found, chances are they will label you as a pill popper, attention seeker or even as far as "it is all in the mind".

I am sure a lot of us can relate to this behaviour from the medical profession.

# All the Multiple Sclerosis symptoms

I have covered about five symptoms in the previous chapter, so let us explore the rest.

**Paresthesia** will in most cases develop in to Paresis, severely affecting your balance and walking in the later years of Multiple Sclerosis, and in patients with severe MS, the use of the effected limb may be lost forever. Paresthesia is a sensation of tickling, tingling, burning, pricking, or numbness of a person's skin with no apparent long-term physical effect. The main symptoms are the feeling of "Pins and Needles" for no apparent reason. The feeling is similar to a limb falling asleep. Paresthesia of the hands and feet are common however transient symptoms of the related conditions can lead to hyperventilation syndrome, and panic attacks.

This symptom of Multiple Sclerosis is one that most people seek help for, as it is so common and it is clear that it is a neurological. It feels like:

- Numbness

- Pins and needles

- Burning

- Severe itchiness

- Tingling, buzzing, vibrating sensations

Paresthesia in Multiple Sclerosis is caused by lesions on the brain or spinal cord. It is sometimes set off by something touching the limb or they can occur spontaneously. It normally starts in the hands and feet and then moves upwards. This symptom is very frustrating and is also affected by external factors such as heat tolerance and MS fatigue.

**Paresis** is the loss of use of muscles which will eventually develop atrophy. It comes from the ancient Greek words "Letting Go" or paralysis "to let go, to let fall." Paresis is an advanced sign of MS and is commonly seen in patients with progressive Multiple Sclerosis. Paresis leads to further muscle stiffness or atrophy due to mild or partial paresis of the muscle. In the beginning stage of paresis the muscle may tremor or spasm. Involuntary jerking movements also present themself in the patient. One of the most known symptoms of muscle control loss is the so called restless leg syndrome which occurs when the patient's legs are resting, mostly at night when you are trying to sleep. Spasticity is normal in the above with the muscle being stiff or in spasm due to paresis of the muscle. In severe cases of MS these spasms can actually cause a MS patient to violently jerk leading to extreme pain. Also present in the above group can be bladder and bowel problems, with frequent visits to the toilet or the inability to control the bladder movement.

This is the most debilitating symptom of Multiple Sclerosis and is also the most feared. The more the progression in Multiple Sclerosis affects you the worse it becomes. Losing one's ability to walk is not for the fainthearted and is especially challenging.

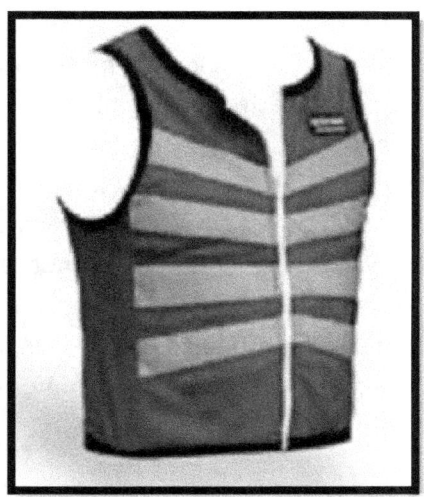

[43] Cooling Vest (Image courtesy of Arctic Heat USA)

Environmental factors play a huge role in Paresis, with heat being the most common one. MS patients tend to not do too well in heat. Any temperature above the average cool range can affect us very badly, as the hotter it gets the worst the Paresis or numbness gets. Temporary relief from heat can be found in a good air conditioned home keeping the temperature around 22° Celsius or 72° Fahrenheit. Simple cooler vest can also be worn to lower the body core temperature.

On the next symptom I am going to dwell a bit, as this affects a MS patient quite badly and is their major symptom.

**Ataxia** is caused by the patient's inability to walk properly and has a loss of balance control and coordination. Foot drop is also a sign of Ataxia where the patient has problems controlling his feet or the foot drops uncontrollably during walking, leading to spectacular falls.  Posture problems are also reported. In most cases the patient does not stand in a proper manner and the one side of the body is bending either sideways or forward. The patient also has a problem picking up or moving objects. In severe cases the patient may appear "drunk". Ataxia consists of lack of voluntary coordination of muscle movements and is a sign of a neurological dysfunction of  the cerebellum in the brain. In other words lesions or plaques in the motor movement part of the brain.

Think of it as a telephone signal loss. Your brain is in constant communication with your limbs etc. When that communication gets disrupted or delayed you will see the effect. A simple thing like walking, a daily task that normal people take for granted can become a daunting task. Foot drop is a good example. The muscle to move and lift the foot is there, however the telephone line from the brain to the foot is not functioning properly. In essence the brain tells the leg to lift, as we are now going walking. This part functions normally, but the foot somehow loses the message. So as you set merrily along your way, your foot, by not lifting properly, may drop, thus causing you to trip and fall over your own foot. You will notice patients with severe MS will tend to walk at a slow pace with the foot or feet dragging on the ground or close by. The foot is not in the normal position but in a hanging situation. There are numerous devices designed to combat this symptom and are available to you.

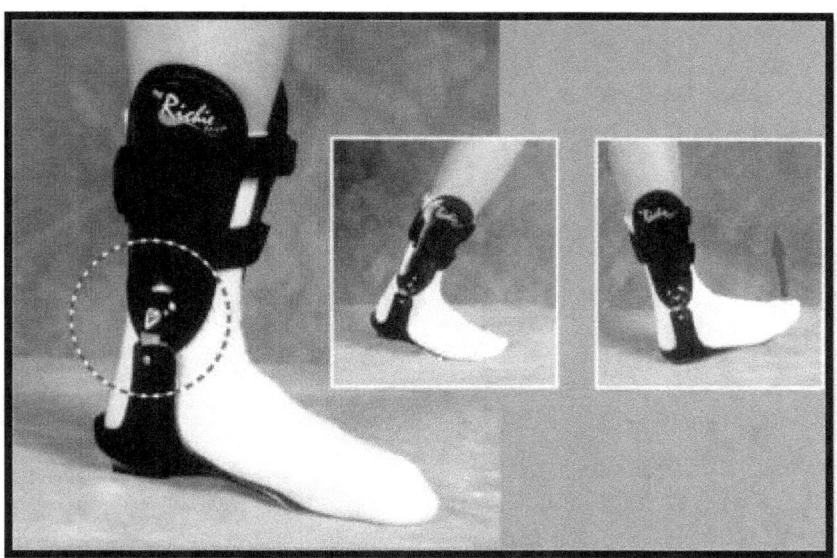

[44] Foot Drop Brace. (Image courtesy of Richie Technologies Inc.)

**Gait Ataxia** is another symptom of MS and also falls under Ataxia. Gait Ataxia is the primary cause of imbalance in Multiple Sclerosis. This primarily caused by lesion in the cerebellum or the Latin for "little brain"

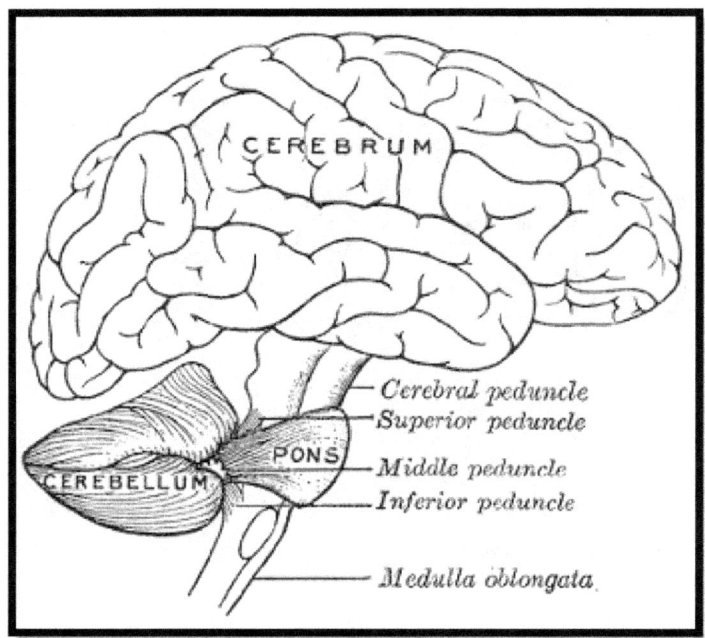

[45] The little brain or Cerebellum (Image source: Wikipedia)

The cerebellum is the motor control centre of the brain and is responsible for balance, co-ordination, timing and accuracy. Certain other functions are also performed by this little brain. Cognitive functions such as attention and language, and the regulating of fear and pleasure responses is controlled here as well. However the spinal cord can also play a big part in Gait Ataxia. If you present with lesions on the spinal cord it can severely affect your gait, and it is very true of Devic's Disease. The technical term for this is Neuromyelitis optica (NMO is also a form of MS only more severe with the spinal cord and optical nerves affected the most.

There are a couple of tests to see if you do suffer from gait problems. Ever wondered why a neurologist swings your body by the shoulder, or pushes you backwards. In the body swing, you will tend to step backwards to steady your posture, or in pushing, you will lose a bit of balance trying to steady yourself. This is to determine if you have a normal gait. Any abnormal gait movements are detected in this way. Then there is also the ten metres heal to toe walk with or without head turns. The finger to the nose test or finger to finger test is also applied. Any abnormalities to a normal gait can be determined by these tests. Trust me I got stopped in a roadblock once and asked to walk heal to toe. I had to carefully explain I was not drunk, but that I have Multiple Sclerosis.

**Sensory Ataxia** is also characterised under Ataxia. Sensory Ataxia is mainly caused by a loss of sensory input in control and movement. This will affect a MS Patient as you never know which part of your body is where or what it is touching. Sensory ataxia is tested by a couple of quick tests. Once again the finger to the nose however this time, with your eyes closed. Another one is the Romberg's test. Again the walking test is applied comprising of the heel to toe test, also noting whether any unusual stomping of the feet is present. The arms are extended to the physician in a ninety degree position to the body with the eyes closed. Any drifting down of the fingers and or sudden jerking back is a positive Romberg sign.

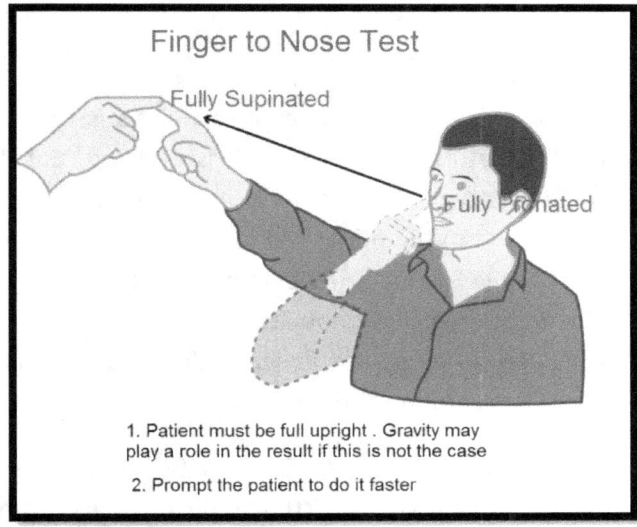

[46] Finger to Nose test (Image courtesy of Grant Groenenstein)

Sensory ataxia is a direct cause of proprioceptive dis-function. In this test you are requested to close your eyes. With the absence of sight, the body is unaware where the limb is and cannot interpret its position to movement. Generally this is caused by dysfunction of the dorsal columns of the spinal cord. This is caused by the lack of ability to carry proprioceptive information to the brain. Other causes of sensory ataxia can be a dysfunction of the various parts of the brain which receive positional information, including the cerebellum, thalamus, and parietal lobes.

If you can pass these tests you might still be fine to drive. Failing these might land you in trouble with the law and you will have to do some serious explanations.

**Dysarthria** is a speech disorder found in Multiple Sclerosis and primarily caused by neuromuscular impairment, which results in loss of motor control of the speech mechanism. The demyelinating lesions caused by Multiple Sclerosis may result in spasticity, weakness, slowness, and/or ataxic incoordination of the lips, tongue, mandible, soft palate, vocal cords, and diaphragm. It involves the muscle that we need to talk, and can make it difficult to pronounce words properly. The cranial nerves are mostly affected. These include the trigeminal nerve motor branch, the facial nerve, glossopharyngeal nerve as well as the vagus nerve. The cranial we have dealt with under Trigeminal Neuralgia. The glossopharyngeal and vagus nerve exit the brain at the same spot as the cranial nerve.

Word articulation is one of the most affected parts of later stages or advanced MS. Slurred speech forms part of this pattern as well as slow speech. This is typical indication of speech involvement. The natural flow of speech is affected, but it does not mean that the cognitive function of the patient is impaired. The slow pallet impaired speech is directly the result of the muscle needed for speech being compromised. Typical in advanced Multiple Sclerosis, the person is perceived to be drunk and coupled with that if there is a walking disability, makes you want to shout "I am not drunk, I have MS". Certain drugs like epileptic drugs, commonly used in MS to treat certain pain types, can compromise speech further.

Studies point to speech disorders ranging from 23% to as high as 51%, however this is not a clear indication of the exact figures as most studies on this vary from country to country. Treatment at a speech therapist can certainly benefit some patients.

**Dysphonia** often accompanies Dysarthria. This is more a type of voice disorder with pitch, loudness and nasal resonance being affected. Voice quality is also impaired due to paresis of one or both sides of the larynx.

**Dysarthria and dysphonia** in MS may be accompanied by the underlying symptoms of spasticity, weakness, tremor and ataxia; and complicated by fatigue. Fatigue can worsen the affect Multiple Sclerosis can have on your speech. Remember; a MS patient's cognitive function remains intact the longest, so if we speak slowly "We are not mentally retarded, we are just having trouble speaking".

**Dysphagia** or difficulty in swallowing is quite common in Multiple Sclerosis with between 30-40% affected by this. Dysphagia can be very mild in some patient, but also so severe that some might need a feeding tube later on. In the advance stages of Multiple Sclerosis this might be all too real. Swallowing is mostly controlled by the brainstem or the Medulla Oblongata and Pons, the part of the brain that controls autonomic functions. The Brain stem is the connection between the spinal cord and brain. Lesions in this area can cause Dysphagia.

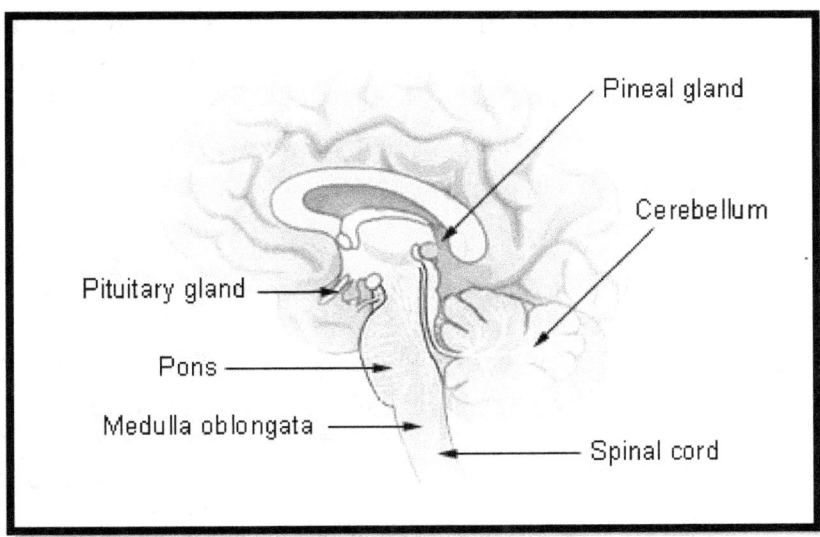

[47] Brain Stem, Medulla Oblongata and Pons (Image source: Wikipedia)

Some Multiple Sclerosis patients do not even realize that they suffer from Dysphagia as it can be so subtle that they experience it as food or drink going down the wrong pipe i.e. the breathing path. Several factors play a leading role in swallowing problems. The most common is a delay in pharyngeal swallowing. The pharynx and Oesophagus is the actual throat pipe to the stomach, and it contracts and relaxes in the process of swallowing. Swallowing excess saliva (common in most patients) and liquids is the first signs of dysphagia. The simple swallowing of a vitamin or painkillers can become a problem, and I for one, suffer from it.

A reduced Pharynx or Oesophagus wall contraction is also a problem in Dysphagia. Weakness caused by the pharynx or Oesophageal wall muscle causes swallowing problems too. So just as in the muscle in the legs and arms, the throat muscles are also affected by Multiple Sclerosis. This type of Dysphagia causes mostly food to remain in the windpipe long after we have swallowed it.

A sign of Dysphagia includes difficult chewing, excessive saliva, drooling, choking or the feeling that the food is difficult to swallow. Coughing directly after swallowing is very common in Dysphagia, but also a very real indicator of more serious problems that may follow. Aspiration pneumonia is typical in Dysphagia. Aspiration pneumonia is caused by tiny food particles landing up in the bronchial track of the lungs. These small particles cause infection in the lung, which in turn leads to pneumonia. Vomiting can also happen after eating and causes not only food particles but also stomach acid landing in the lungs. To a certain extent, lack of saliva or a dry mouth can worsen it. Some of the drugs we take have these side effects.

A couple of treatments are available for this. Treatment consisting mainly of anti-epileptic drugs is the main one and as well as some anti-depressants.

A physician can test for Dysphagia, but this is not a great test to go through and is probably one of the most uncomfortable. A tube gets inserted through the nasal passage into the throat and pressure readings upon swallowing are measured. It is called an Oesophagus Manometer Test. Barium x-ray testing can also show food being lodged in the pharynx or Oesophagus during the process of swallowing. Barium is a liquid that acts as a contrast enhancer for normal x-rays, and will show up in the x-ray.

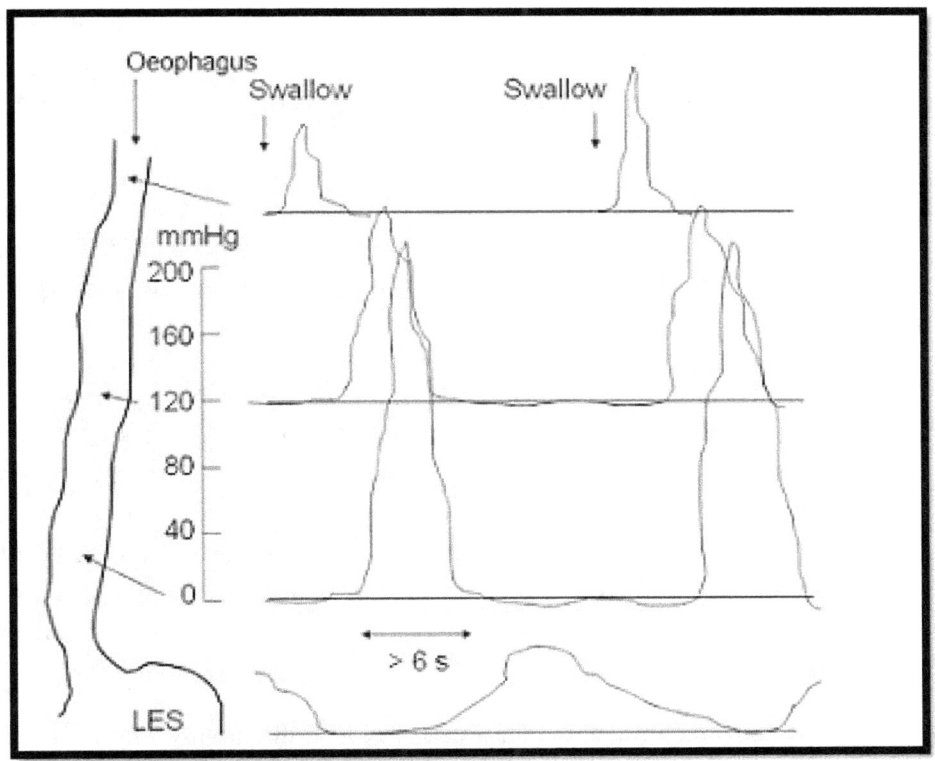

[48] Oesophagus Manometer Test (Source: Wikipedia. Author: Samir)

Gastroesophageol reflux (GERD) or difficulty swallowing is not uncommon in Multiple Sclerosis. GERD is caused primarily by the sphincter (Stomach valve) in the diaphragm not functioning properly. The cause of this is normally a lesion in the brain-stem involving the 10 cranial nerve (Vagus nerve or wandering nerve). The sphincter can be compromised in two ways. The first is the sphincter not opening enough causing difficulty in swallowing. This is referred to as Dysphagia in Multiple Sclerosis. This is normally caused by either a spastic diaphragm muscle or the sphincter itself being spastic.

The second effect is caused by the sphincter not closing properly. This also cause reflux in the oesophagus causing gastric fluid leaking back into the oesophagus. Heartburn is normally the first indication of this. In certain severe cases it also causes a Hiatal hernia. A Hiatal hernia is a part of the stomach protruding through the diaphragm. This is caused by a dysfunction in the sphincter. Another complication of GERD is Aspiration Pneumonia. This is caused by small particles of foods or stomach acid landing in the lungs, causing a lung infection which leads to pneumonia. This is very often seen at the higher scale of disability and normally in patients that are in frail care. It is a major complication of end stages of Multiple Sclerosis.

**Neuropathic pain** results from damage or disease affecting the sensory system. Some neuropathic pain is directly associated with the area of pain in Optic Neuritis and Trigeminal Neuralgia. However, in high percentage, this is directly associated with the damage of the trigeminal nerve and optic nerves.

The vast majority of neuropathic pain is associated with influencing our daily lives. Neuropathic pain, in short, is a pain that is actually not present at the area of the pain, but is caused by damage to the brain or spinal cord nerves. Neuropathic pain is considered a pain syndrome instead of an actual pain. There's a big misconception that the "Pain is all in the Head", which in fact is actually true, but this lead to some doctors dismissing the actual pain complaint in Multiple Sclerosis. This may lead to some doctors erroneously to dismiss your pain. In reality, you are definitely experiencing pain

Today this pain syndrome is very common in MS and is now being recognised by most doctors. A study done on pain in MS suggests that as much as 55% of people with MS had "clinically significant pain" at some time. This study suggested that factors such as age at onset, length of time with MS, or degree of disability played no role in differentiating MS patient's pain from those who were pain free. A clear indication from this study shows that this pain type is found more often in women than men.

The pain symptoms are burning, itching, wetness, girdling affects and pins and needles and are neurological in origin, in other words, it is the head, but it is very real pain and can be devastating to some MS patients. The pain can be constant or experienced as short bursts of pain, like an electric jolt. The technical term for this is Dysesthesias and comes from the Greek word "dys", meaning "not-normal" and "aesthesis", which means "sensation". In plain English it is not a normal sensation, and is caused by lesions of the nervous system in the brain and spine. This pain is mostly treated and controlled by anti-convulsion drugs (Epileptics) and anti-depressants. Relief may also be found by wearing pressure stockings, gloves that assist in converting to a sensation of pressure instead of pain. Warm compresses to the skin can also relieve this pain to a certain extend.

**Lhermitte's sign** is a common symptom in Multiple Sclerosis and also classified as neuropathic pain. Lhermitte's sign was describe by Jean Lhermite in 1920, a French doctor specialising in nervous system diseases. The presence of lesions in the spinal cord in the upper spine area below the brain is mostly the cause of this. He did studies on MS patients who suffered from so-called electrical shocks sensation in the spine that shoots to the limbs when they move or flex their necks forward and backwards. However, it was first noted by Marie Chatelin in 1917. It is also known as the Barber Chair phenomenon. As with other neuropathic pain, epileptic drugs are used to control this. Wearing a soft collar can also help to reduce the flexing of the neck. Studies indicate that 38% of all MS patient experience this type of pain.

Lhermitte's sign is not specific to MS. It is a symptom that can occur with any abnormality of the cervical spinal cord, usually involving active inflammation or impingement on a disc. It can occur with vitamin B12 deficiency, cervical spondylitis, and other conditions. An MRI may be required to rule out other possible causes.

**Myoclonus** is a brief jerking of a muscle or a group of muscle. Myoclonus comes from the Greek words "Myo" meaning "muscle" and "Clonus" meaning "tumult", describing the sudden and uncontrollable shock-like movements or "jerks" of a muscle or a group of muscles. Myoclonus is caused by contractions and relaxation of muscles. Myoclonus appears mainly at rest or while you are in the process of falling asleep. Myoclonus can also cause hiccups in certain patients, especially if the diaphragm muscle is involved. It may appear in a pattern or without a pattern. The occurrence can be short and infrequent or span over several times per minute.

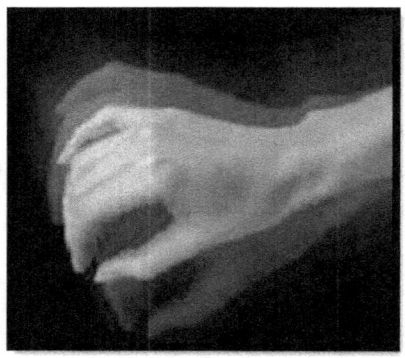

[49] Typical myoclonus jerking. (Image courtesy of anonymous patient)

The onset of myoclonus usually indicates a lesion in the cortex, sub cortex or the spinal cord. Myoclonus can be mild to so severe that it can disrupt the patient's everyday life. The treatment for myoclonus is clonazepam or bensodiasepam. This is only prescribed when myoclonus is severe in the patient as these drugs can be addictive. Due to the complexities of Myoclonus it may prove necessary to use more than one drug to provide an effective treatment, and doctors may combine several drugs together to control the Myoclonus jerks. Myoclonus is more frequent during the night than in daytime.

**Restless Leg Syndrome (RLS)** or Wittmaack-Ekbom's syndrome is characterised by MS patient to involuntarily move the legs in a shaking or jerking manner. Normally this is sub conscious and you don't realise it happening. Restless leg syndrome is five times more prevalent in MS patients than the norm in healthy individuals with about 10-15% being affected. It may also affect other parts of the body like the hands and arms but is mostly subjected to the legs. RLS is caused by a burning, itching or pins and needles sensation in the affected body parts. The sensation can be so mild that it is not noticeable but may still cause RLS. It is a voluntary response of the body to get rid of this sensation. RLS typically begins or intensifies during quiet wakefulness, such as when relaxing, reading, studying, or trying to sleep. RLS is classified as a Myoclonus jerk, and in patients who have limb jerking during sleep, it falls under the term nocturnal Myoclonus. RLS in children is often misdiagnosed as growing pains and could be an early indicator of Multiple Sclerosis later on in life, although this is not yet confirmed.

Sir Thomas Willis first noted the description of RLS in 1672. The first description read: "Wherefore to some, when being abed they betake themselves to sleep, presently in the arms and legs, leaping's and contractions on the tendons, and so great a restlessness and

tossing's of other members ensue, that the diseased are no more able to sleep, than if they were in a place of the greatest torture."

The best description in early medical literature was by Theodur Wittmaack (1861) and in 1945 Karl-Axel Ekbom (1907–1977) provided a detailed and comprehensive report of this condition in his doctoral thesis, "Restless legs: clinical study of hitherto overlooked diseases". This led to the term Wittmaack-Ekbom's syndrome. His clinical notes were based on Parkinson's and related diseases but today this is a familiar symptom in MS.

A Mild sedative may help in this case or a muscle relaxant. RLS is not noticed when the patient is active but more active when the patient is in rest. An anticonvulsant may help but could in some cases worsen RLS. Walking the feeling off can help in most cases. In MS patients, it can be from a slight inconvenience to a major disruption. Recent Medical studies have indicated that RLS may be an early warning sign of Multiple Sclerosis. Although RLS is disrupting, it is not a severe symptom. In the case where it affects the natural sleeping pattern it will have an effect on the Fatigue pertaining to Multiple Sclerosis.

**Uveitis and phlebitis** is more commonly found in Multiple Sclerosis patients, than in normal persons. This could sometimes be seen as an early symptom of Multiple Sclerosis or a flare up of Multiple Sclerosis. Uveitis specifically refers to inflammation of the middle layer of the eye, termed the "uvea". Uveitis is inflammation of the middle layer of the eye. The classical symptoms are blurred vision, redness and painful eyes. Classic markers are dark spots floating around in the eyes or light sensitivity. In Multiple Sclerosis patients, the inflammation in normally in the posterior chamber of the eye, in other words the small space between the Iris and the lens. Uveitis in Multiple Sclerosis is a classic sign of an immune response in the body. Normally accompanying uveitis is Optic Neuritis. This is in most cases a classical symptom of a flare up in Multiple Sclerosis.

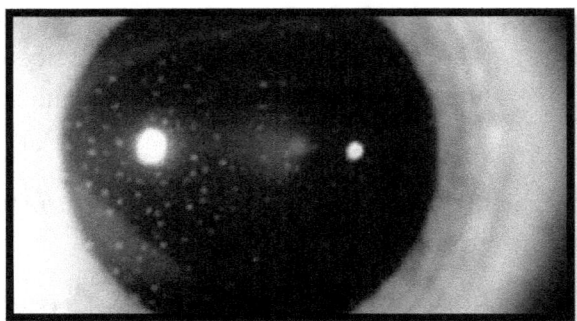

[50] Anterior granulomatous uveitis in a patient with multiple sclerosis. (Source: National Library of Medicine (NLM))

**Phlebitis** normally accompanies the above condition. Phlebitis is inflammation of the small veins in the eye and on the eyeball itself. Thus the eye appears very red and is highly irritated and painful. In severe case of phlebitis of the eye, there can be small haemorrhages of the small veins in the eye. The lesion that forms in the case of uveitis and retinal phlebitis is similar to the lesions that form in the Central Nervous System.

The normal treatment for this will be steroid drops and oral prednisone or in case of a Multiple Sclerosis flare up; an IV steroid course is recommended. Uveitis is a leading course of blindness in the USA and if left untreated in Multiple Sclerosis, can lead to blindness.

**Vertigo or dizziness** is present in about 20% of Multiple Sclerosis patients. This is the sensation of the roof spinning or you spinning in the room. The most common of it all is when you lie down and you get the feeling that the room is spinning around you or drifting/tilting away from you. Another feeling is the feeling of the ground coming up to meet you. This is a common symptom of Multiple Sclerosis. The sensation is short lasting but can carry on in bouts for weeks on end. It can sometimes get so bad that you get dizzy or vomit from this.

The most common causes of this can be two fold. The one is a lesion in the cerebellum, the part of the brain that controls motion or movement. The other can be due to a lesion in the brain stem, particularly the nerve that controls the function of the ear. However it is also true that in MS patients it can be due to benign paroxysmal position vertigo. This is caused by crystals in our ears that move to the wrong position in the ear and can be painlessly repaired by a GP. Over the counter meds for inner ear imbalance can also help.

The roll test can be done to determine whether the horizontal semi-circular ear canal is involved. The test requires the patient to be in a laying down position with the face up, with his/her head in 20° of forward flexion. The head is rotated 90° to the left side, and examiner checks for vertigo and nystagmus. This is followed by gently bringing the head back to the starting position. The test is then repeated to the other side. In the roll test, you may experience vertigo and nystagmus on both sides, but the affected side will trigger a more intense vertigo. Similarly, when the head is rotated towards the affected side, the nystagmus will beat towards the ground and be more intense

**Nystagmus** is a form of involuntary eye movements in MS patient. The main feature of it is the normal smooth movement of the eyes in one direction and a jerking movement in the opposite direction while tracking an object with the eyes. Nystagmus can even happen while you are watching something and the eyes tend to jerk, causing the object to jerk or blur in front of you. Standard test for this is to have the patient track an object from left to right. It can be mild to severe in Multiple Sclerosis patient.

There are two forms of nystagmus in Multiple Sclerosis. The one is vestibular nystagmus, due to balance problems as a result of the auditory centre in the brain being affected by Multiple Sclerosis. The second is central nystagmus, due to lesions in the mid brain or cerebellum. Central nystagmus also causes up and down jerking of one or both eyes. There is no cure for this; however Baclofen and Gabapentin bring some relief to patents with this symptom.

**Pseudo Bulbar Affect (PBA)** is a condition in Multiple Sclerosis and may be known by other names including "emotional incontinence" or "Involuntary Emotional Expression Disorder." Basically it means that you may have bouts of uncontrollable laughing or crying without feeling the emotions associated with your expression. You might start crying but really be feeling content. You may begin to laugh without warning and without finding anything funny. Once the person starts to cry or laugh they may find it nearly impossible to stop. This is frequent in 10% of MS Patients and can also be a first symptom of MS. PBA is generally associated with later stages of the disease especially in the progressive stage. PBA in MS patients is associated with more severe intellectual impairment, physical disability, and mental dysfunction.

The symptoms of PBA can be severe, with persistent and unremitting episodes including the following:

- Onset can be sudden and unpredictable, and has been described by some patients as coming on like a seizure;

- Outbursts have a typical duration of a few seconds to several minutes; and,

- Outbursts may happen several times a day.

Some antidepressants may be helpful in decreasing the symptoms of PBA (pseudo bulbar affect). There are medications which have been used in some clinical trials and was found to be beneficial in treating PBA include: Amitriptyline, Levodopa, Desipramine, Fluoxetine, and Fluvoxamine. The above in low dosages seem to help for it.

Avanir Pharmaceuticals are looking into further studies of a medication called Zenvia, which is taken orally. Zenvia should be approved in a couple of months.

**Uhtoff's Phenomenon** is experienced when hot weather, saunas and warm baths can cause your MS symptoms to worsen. Also on hot days, you feel more fatigue than normal. This syndrome was first observed in 1890 by Wilhelm Uhtoff in patients with Optic Neuritis. Thus it became known as the Uhtoff's syndrome. In a later study pertaining to damage to the Central Nervous Symptom it was observed that similar effects were present.

Peripheral nerve studies have shown that even a 0.5°C increase in body temperature can slow or block the conduction of nerve impulses in demyelinated nerves. With greater levels of demyelination, a smaller increase in temperature is needed to slow down the nerve impulse conduction. Exercising and performing activities of daily living can cause a significant increase in body temperature in individuals with MS, especially if their mechanical efficiency is poor due to the use of mobility aids, ataxia, weakness, and spasticity. However, exercise has been shown to be helpful in managing MS symptoms, reducing the risk of comorbidities, and promoting overall wellness.

Multiple Sclerosis sufferers should avoid exposure to heat as it can exacerbate the symptoms. The same is true for exercise, as this increases the body's core temperature.

**Fatigue** is probably the most debilitating symptom of Multiple Sclerosis. The majority of Multiple Sclerosis patients suffer from this, and this symptom does not disappear even sometimes when they are in relapse. Between 80-95% of all Multiple Sclerosis patients are affected by MS fatigue. This symptom in most MS patients is ever present in their lives. The fatigue in most cases takes on two forms, one being mental fatigue which is highly prevalent in MS. The other being physical fatigue, where the body is affected and the symptom of this are fatigue with movement and motion.

Researchers are beginning to outline the characteristics of this so-called "MS fatigue" that make it different from fatigue experienced by persons without MS.

- Generally occurs on a daily basis

- May occur early in the morning, even after a restful night's sleep

- Tends to worsen as the day progresses

- Tends to be aggravated by heat and humidity

- Comes on easily and suddenly

- Is generally more severe than normal fatigue

- Is more likely to interfere with daily responsibilities

**Mental fatigue** is present in a daily pattern, where the patient feels the need to rest as they are mentally exhausted. This varies from patient to patient and is sometimes mild to severe. MS Patients are known to need rest periods during the day and to take naps to overcome this fatigue. Mental fatigue can also be exacerbated by heat and a raise in the body's core temperature (Uhtoff's phenomenon). This type of fatigue is also more severe in PPMS and SPMS patient, with the level of fatigue increasing as the disease progresses. Mental fatigue is also related to depression in Multiple Sclerosis. Mental fatigue levels normally increase as the day progresses. A short nap or total rest during the day when the fatigue sets in seems to help the patient.

**Physical fatigue** is easily experienced after short walks or exercise. Physical fatigue involves the body's ability to handle physical activity. This definitely follows the disease patterns, in other words, the more the progression the more the fatigue. For some reason, also not fully understood, the efficiency of demyelinised nerves deteriorates very rapidly with use. Almost everyone whose physical functioning has been disturbed through MS finds that their ability to do things reduces as they do them. In Multiple Sclerosis, walking can feel like running a marathon as walking is in most case a very exhaustive task. As with mental fatigue and most other MS symptoms, heat makes physical fatigue worse. Exercise can also raise the body's core temperature leading to this fatigue being increased.

Fatigue in MS appears not to be unrelated to disability status, and many patients complain of fatigue even when all their other symptoms are mild or in complete remission. This fatigue is not fully understand but sleep disturbances, could be caused by restless leg syndrome or urinary patterns at the night. Pain at night time interfering with sleep can also be a factor in this fatigue. There is no direct correlation between lesion load and position of the lesions and fatigue. However lesions in the cerebellum and brainstem that cause involuntary night time spasms are implicated. MS-related fatigue does not appear to be directly correlated with either depression or the degree of physical impairment.

Certain Biomarkers found in MS patients could be an aggravating factor. Creatine and Uric acid levels are lower than normal, especially in female Multiple Sclerosis patients. Creatine is nitrogenous organic acid that occurs naturally in humans and helps to supply energy to muscles. Creatine is naturally produced in the human body from amino acids primarily in the kidney and liver. It is transported in the blood for use by muscles. At least 95% of the human body's total Creatine is located in muscle. The rest is located in the brain or heart. This reduction in Creatine could lead to the chronic fatigue symptoms in MS Patients.

Treatments for fatigue are symptomatic, and are mainly treated with Amantadine, Modafinil, Pemoline, Methylphenidate and Provigil. The new theory CCSVI and the treatment of balloon angioplasty do indicate strongly to help with this fatigue. What effect this has on fatigue still needs to be clearly understood.

**Headaches** are common in Multiple Sclerosis patients, and we are much more prone to cluster or migraine headaches than the normal population. Current figures put this close to 60 % of Multiple Sclerosis patients, substantially more than the 16% of normal people. Most people get a headache from time to time but the type describes below is different than normal headaches.

The most common type that most of us know is the headaches that accompany Optic Neuritis. The first sign of Optic Neuritis is a cluster like headache which is associated to one side of the face. This headache is normally associated with a painful eye movements or stabbing pains behind the eye. It can be so bad that the patient can complain of tears in the eyes. Headaches can also appear in people with trigeminal neuralgia. In certain cases patient experience these cluster headaches but without any signs of Optic Neuritis or trigeminal neuralgia.  Most of the times this is cluster headaches and is restricted to the side where there is a neuropathic pain. These cluster headaches can cause the eyes to water or the nose to run. It also causes the eyelids to droop. This type of headache sometimes comes without any warning and can last for hours.

Multiple Sclerosis patients with definite lesions in the part of the mid brain where the cranial nerve exits the brain are more prone to suffer from cluster headaches. Although there is **no** definite connection with these flare ups and headaches, many a patient will attest to it.

Certain medication that we, as Multiple Sclerosis patients, are prescribed can also cause headaches. Most of the interferon range of medication has headaches as common side effects. Some of the medicine that we use to treat fatigue like Provigil can lead to an increase of headaches. The above headaches are mild and not as frequent as the headaches that are involved with Optic Neuritis.

Low serotonin levels in Multiple Sclerosis patients can also lead to headaches. They suffer more from migraine headaches. A drop in Serotonin levels can lead to depression and migraine headaches.

Another cause for headaches in Multiple Sclerosis patients is due to intracranial hypertension, in other words the increase of brain fluid in the brain. There is still no clear link between Multiple Sclerosis and increase intracranial hypertension. It has been indicated in several studies that Multiple Sclerosis lesions in the brain can lead to higher intracranial pressure, similar to tumours in the brain. These headaches, due to increase intracranial pressure, can be very severe leading to nausea, dizziness, double vision and slurred speech. Some patients have reported similar symptoms as a patient with a head injury that has caused this increased intracranial pressure. Research has still not clearly identified the increase of intracranial pressure as an onset of a Multiple Sclerosis flare-up, however there are strong indications that this may be the fact. That there is a definite increase in intracranial pressure in some Multiple Sclerosis is a fact. Whether MS flare-up causes increase intracranial pressure or increase intracranial pressure causes a MS flare-up is still a mystery.

Still not to be excluded, is the fact that the Steroid treatment can also lead to intracranial pressure. This can also lead to headaches during and after steroid treatment.

**Hearing problems** are also present in Multiple Sclerosis but is a relatively unspoken topic. Similar to Optic Neuritis the connection between the inner ear and the brain can also be affected by MS. In 85% of MS patients that do suffer from hearing loss it was found that their ability to hear higher frequency tone is impaired. The problem may be only limited to one ear or can effect both ears. Some patients may even suffer a sudden hearing loss when they are in relapse with improvement when they are in remission.

So to put it in a nutshell, the hearing impairment is normally in the higher auditory tract, affecting the eighth auditory nerve. In other words, the higher tones being heard as a lower tone, and for this reason some MS patients have difficulty hearing when there is background noise present as their normal auditory tract is affected and the brain has difficulty processing the difference in the low frequency and high frequency noise . In some MS patients, this hearing problem was present before any other symptoms. Brainstem Auditory Evoked Potentials (BAEPs), a test to determine if there is any hearing function loss is done today in most MS patients. This test, a means to measure auditory nerve function is widely used in today by all MS specialists.

Some Multiple Sclerosis patients may also suffer from Tinnitus, a ringing or buzzing noise in the ear. However, Tinnitus is a very common side effect of the wide range of medication that is used to treat Multiple Sclerosis and the wide range of symptoms. Please note that there are not a lot of studies on this, but I did discover some studies.

**Sexual dysfunction** in Multiple Sclerosis is a subject that is rarely covered and often overlooked. The sad reality is this is very real symptom and a marriage breaker. In describing sexual dysfunction we tend to categorise only males, with the tools of the trade not working, but it affects women just as badly as men.

Studies have shown that 63% of patients indicated that their sexual activity had declined since having Multiple Sclerosis. About 90% of male patients are affected by this, and in the case of woman the figure is as high as 70%. It is however rarely discussed between doctors and patients, due to the nature of the topic. About 40% of all Multiple Sclerosis patients tend to stop their sexual activity al together.

In women, symptoms include:

- Reduced sensation in the vaginal and clitoral area, or painfully heightened sensation

- Vaginal dryness

- Difficulty achieving orgasm

- Loss of libido

In men, symptoms include:

- Difficulty achieving or maintaining an erection is by far the most common problem

- Reduced sensation in the penis

- Difficulty achieving orgasm or ejaculation

- Loss of libido

Fatigue can play a major part in sexual dysfunction, and the "Honey not now I am tired" has certainly been thrown around in the bedroom. Emotion can play a big role in this as well. As with any disease of this magnitude there are certain feelings of low self-esteem, anxiety, anger and depression. Your mental well-being plays an important role in this aspect.

Sexual dysfunction has many causes and effects in Multiple Sclerosis, including blood circulation problems, hormonal state and nerve functioning. Lesions in the brain can interfere with the sexual stimuli function in the brain, while lesions in the spinal cord could ultimately block or reduce the signal to the components of the body to engage in such acts.

This does not need to be a "Marriage breaker", as in today's modern world there are many forms of treatments for this problem. My first suggestion is, if you feel uncomfortable talking to your doctor about it, go and see a sex therapist or marriage counsellor. There are also many options available medical-wise, that I will deal with here instead of the chapter dealing with medication.

For the men, erectile dysfunction may be addressed through use of the oral medications Viagra, Levitra, and Cialis. There are also injectable medications such as Papaverine and Phentolamine that increase blood flow in the "soldier" to get him to attention. However I would prefer the pill option rather than injecting my "soldier". Another form of treatment is the MUSE system which involves inserting a small suppository into the "soldier". The option of implanted inflatable devices can also be used as a last resort.

Women experiencing vaginal dryness, pain or burning; oestrogen creams may be useful. A vaginal suppository cream is another treatment for these symptoms, although this form may not be available in all countries. There are also a few over the counter creams that may be purchased at the drugstore, or even at an adult store.

The lack of sexual drive and performance does not need to kill romance. There are major amounts of vitamins and libido enhancers like ginseng tablets that will help. The best advice is to speak to your partner and discuss the option before this symptom becomes a reality in your bedroom. Do not allow Multiple Sclerosis to destroy your marriage and address this problem from the start.

**Charles Bonnet syndrome** in short, is visual hallucinations that are not accompanied by any other psychotic symptoms in individuals that do not have cognitive problems. Although Multiple Sclerosis can sometimes lead to certain mental diseases like bipolar syndrome, depression etc., Charles Bonnet Syndrome is rarely reported in Multiple Sclerosis, but recently certain cases of this have appeared in MS Patients that do not have cognitive impairment.

In one case a 56 year old woman who lost her vision due to Optic Neuritis claimed to see vivid and complicated images. These images changed in shape, colour, and size and included letters and characters including Chinese characters, vegetables, and small animals. And although she knew that these images were not real, they existed at all times, whether she had her eyes open or closed. The woman had Multiple Sclerosis for about 20 years and had no history of any co morbid psychiatric disorders. Besides her temporary loss of vision, she experienced effects on her cervical and thoracic spinal cord. She became bedridden and completely dependent on the care of others. In testing her cognitive functioning, she scored 25 out of 30 points on a Mini-Mental State Examination, and the short come of 5 points were attributed to her visual impairment. In other words, judging from the score she did not have any cognitive impairment. After an MRI of her brain it showed lesions in both periventricular and white matter regions of the lobe of the brain where the visual cortex is situated. After treating her with Carbamazepine treatment the visual hallucinations reduced. However, after she stopped taking Carbamazepine, the visual hallucinations returned, but the hallucinations reduced again taking Carbamazepine.

Charles Bonnet syndrome has been found with advanced age, and patients with cerebral impairment, and visual impairment due to old age as well. But with younger patients with certain diseases involving the eyes and brain, Charles Bonnet syndrome has been reported in the past. Treating the underlying problem caused by the lesions in the visual cortex with Carbamazepine can reduce this symptom in the rare cases where they appear in Multiple Sclerosis. Although Charles Bonnet syndrome is rare in Multiple Sclerosis this phenomenon does happen in cases too when there is cognitive impairment coupled with Optic Neuritis which led to temporary blindness, but is rarely reported as such. But it is underestimated by doctors treating MS as it is sometimes related to the cognitive impairment instead of the visual impairment.

"It is suggested that doctors pay more attention to the nature of hallucinations in order to diagnose Charles Bonnet syndrome, which can be treated effectively with anticonvulsants."

So the next time you have severe Optic Neuritis and see little green men, it is not aliens or too many drugs but rather a symptom of Multiple Sclerosis.

# Mental dysfunction in Multiple Sclerosis

Cognition is part of the higher brain function in human beings. Higher brain functions include memory, behaviour, recognition, speech and actions. Multiple Sclerosis can play a part in affecting your higher brain function. The higher brain function is controlled by three sectors of the brain, these being the frontal lobe, parietal lobe and the temporal lobe. All of these are situated in the cerebrum or cortex as part of the large upper brain structure.

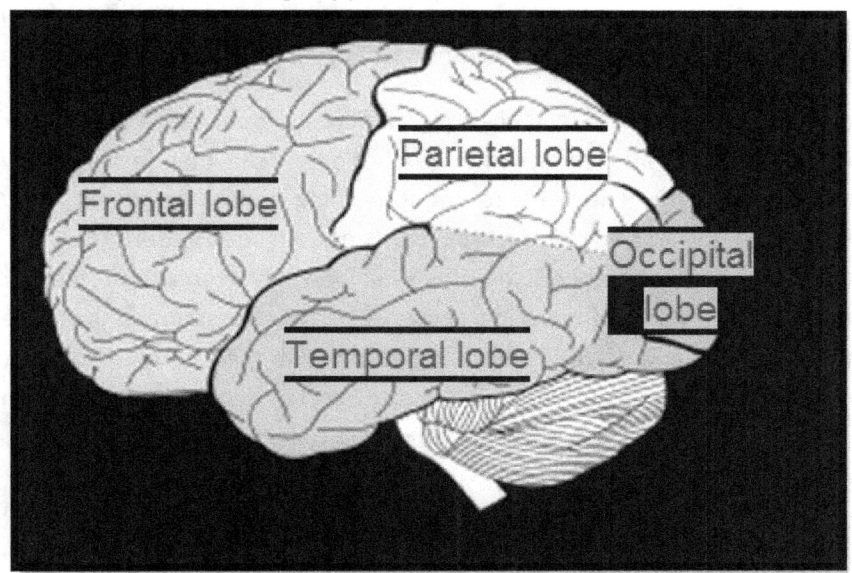

[51] Cerebral Cortex

Symptoms of cognitive dysfunction in Multiple Sclerosis patients are subtle, but in about 5-10%, they are so severe that it will affect their daily lives to such an extent that the person may require care in a specialised facility.

For some of us this feeling is all too familiar. When you dash down to the shops to pick up a desperately needed item, only to arrive home with everything else but the item you went for in the first place. Or you are about to say something in a conversation, and when the moment arrives, you are at a loss for words. You know exactly what you want to say, but somehow the words get lost in the brain somewhere. And then couple that with the inability to function with noise, lights and excessive activity around you, it tends to confuse the thinking part of the brain completely. It can effect certain people to such an extent that they get frozen in the moment, and sends them fleeing from the scene of confusion.

The cognitive functions affected by MS include memory, attention and concentration, the processing of information and executive functions as well as visual perception and constructional abilities stemming from this. Speech or verbal abilities may also be affected.

Multiple Sclerosis patients experience this in many ways and whilst it differs from patient to patient, they all experience it in some form or another.

The effect on the short term memory is the most difficult to deal with. This is by far the most frustrating symptom of Cognitive dysfunction. It can manifest in many different forms. Going to the cupboard to get something only to forget why you went there in the first place. Another example involves your medication. You have just taken your meds and suddenly 5 minutes later you have forgotten whether you have taken them or not.  Repeating sentences in conversation only to be reminded that you just said it, is very frustrating and irritating not only to you, but also to the others in the conversation. This has most certainly been the case with me in writing this book, and believe me, it has not an easy task.

Abstract Conceptualisation, as described in the dictionary, is "to arrive at a concept or generalization as a result of things seen, experienced, or believed". Big words, but this can have a huge impact on Multiple Sclerosis patients in general. MS patients tend to get easily overwhelmed by something that is difficult or complex to understand.  Abstract Conceptualisation means it is hard to organise your thoughts for tasks that a normal healthy person finds easy.  Applying lessons, thoughts and tasks learned from before MS to after MS can be very daunting and difficult. It is very real in people with more advanced forms of Multiple Sclerosis. It can impair your judgement in certain situations to a great extent.

In school we were always taught to be attentive in class, and with good reason. It is something that we take with us and apply to our everyday life.  However, when a medical condition interferes with our attention span, we are disadvantaged and suffer the consequences. Most Multiple Sclerosis patients are easily distracted and the adding of background effects like noise, music or even a television can only worsen this. The simplest task of reading, cooking and day to day tasks can become virtually impossible to complete. Multi-tasking is definitely severely affected.

Taking all of the aforementioned into consideration, our speed and information processes are slowed down. Even processing languages, sensory inputs including smell, touch, sounds and visual information are affected.  The physical location of objects and the metric relationships between objects are distorted with cognitive dysfunction and driving and even walking can be affected.

### So why do we develop cognitive dysfunction?

There are no exact figures as to how many are afflicted with this, however most medical literature puts this figure as high as 65%. The more advanced and aggressive forms of MS show the most prevalence of this. Patients with Secondary Progressive MS are at the top of this scale. Relapsing Remitting MS patient are not as badly affected, but in a relapse these symptoms do tend to appear. However patients with little disability, or in the early stages, can show signs of cognitive dysfunction.

The main contributing factor is brain atrophy, in other words the loss of brain matter due to MS lesions. A T1-weighted magnetic resonance imaging (MRI) scan shows "black holes," which are areas of permanent axonal damage. These are called hypo intense lesions, meaning that they display as dark areas on the MRI image. T1-weighted lesions can also be areas of swelling, which are not permanent and disappear on subsequent scans. Secondary to that, is the presence of lesions in the cerebrum or large brain. Another factor is the axons or nerve endings connecting the left and right brain, being permanently lost due to the destruction of the nerves.

Treatments are symptomatic and can improve cognitive functioning without altering its long-term function. The most successful treatment has been donepezil hydrochloride, showing signs of improvement in verbal memory. This treatment is also used in Alzheimer.

Fatigue plays a huge roll, with metal fatigue the largest. However there are certain drugs that can improve mental as well as physical fatigue. Heat intolerance also affects mental function in Multiple Sclerosis patients.

Depression and Anxiety is common in most MS patients. In most cases this can be due to the effect that MS has on the patient's life and emotional problems arising from MS. However certain studies suggest that anxiety and depression can be a symptom of MS and not due to the patient's mental state.

Yes; your mental state does play a huge role in your life with MS. I am going to elaborate a bit here. Ask any person with a physical disability and at one stage or the other, they went through it or are still dealing with it. The Kübler-Ross model, commonly referred to as the "five stages of grief", names this as the fourth stage in grief. However in Multiple Sclerosis this is a very real stage and normally one of the first as well. Being diagnosed with an incurable disease can lead to a lot of diverse feelings, but the biggest is probably depression.

Depression is an extremely common problem in Multiple Sclerosis. Going from an active normal person to a restricted active lifestyle is not a comfortable feeling, and tends to bring out different emotions in people. Depression interferes with good decision making, relationships and overall functioning thus leading to problems with our day to day functioning as well.

In MS depression may also be a result of the MS disease process itself. Damage to the Myelin and nerve fibres deep within the brain can directly influence your state of mind. Damage that appears in the areas of brain that are involved in emotional expression and control and a variety of behavioural function changes can lead to depression. Depression in MS may also be associated with MS-related changes that occur in the immune and/or neuroendocrine systems. For example, there is some evidence that in persons with MS, changes in mood are accompanied by changes in certain immune parameters

However contrary to logical thought, very severely disabled people are not likely to be more depressed than normal people. Resilience in people plays a big part in this, as we have an extra ordinary ability to adapt to any situation. This is more common in long term MS patients where the progression is slow compared to short term rapid progression.

Severe depression in MS patients does exist and physicians need to note this. The suicide risk among MS patient is 7.5 times higher than usual, and this needs to be addressed before that point is reached. Relapse accounts for an increase in depression and may increase as the disability increases. A side effect of Corticosteroid treatment is depression, and with certain other drugs like interferons as well.

[52] Below is a direct extract from the Kübler-Ross model. (Source: Wikipedia. Author: Elisabeth Kübler-Ross)

-------------------------------------------------------------------------------------

The stages, popularly known by the acronym DABDA, include

Denial — "I feel fine."; "This can't be happening, not to me."

Denial is usually only a temporary defence for the individual. This feeling is generally replaced with heightened awareness of possessions and individuals that will be left behind after death. Denial can be conscious or unconscious refusal to accept facts, information, or the reality of the situation. Denial is a defence mechanism and some people can become locked in this stage.

Anger — "Why me? It's not fair!"; "How can this happen to me?"; '"Who is to blame?"

Once in the second stage, the individual recognizes that denial cannot continue. Because of anger, the person is very difficult to care for due to misplaced feelings of rage and envy. Anger can manifest itself in different ways. People can be angry with themselves, or with others, and especially those who are close to them. It is important to remain detached and non-judgmental when dealing with a person experiencing anger from grief.

Bargaining — "I'll do anything for a few more years."; "I will give my life savings if..."

The third stage involves the hope that the individual can somehow postpone or delay death. Usually, the negotiation for an extended life is made with a higher power in exchange for a reformed lifestyle. Psychologically, the individual is saying, "I understand I will die, but if I could just do something to buy more time..." People facing less serious trauma can bargain or seek to negotiate a compromise. For example "Can we still be friends?" when facing a break-up. Bargaining rarely provides a sustainable solution, especially if it's a matter of life or death.

Depression — "I'm so sad, why bother with anything?"; "I'm going to die soon so what's the point?"; "I miss my loved one, why go on?"

During the fourth stage, the dying person begins to understand the certainty of death. Because of this, the individual may become silent, refuse visitors and spend much of the time crying and grieving. This process allows the dying person to disconnect from things of love and affection. It is not recommended to attempt to cheer up an individual who is in this stage. It is an important time for grieving that must be processed. Depression could be referred to as the dress rehearsal for the 'aftermath'. It is a kind of acceptance with emotional attachment. It's natural to feel sadness, regret, fear, and uncertainty when going through this stage. Feeling those emotions shows that the person has begun to accept the situation.

Acceptance — "It's going to be okay."; "I can't fight it, I may as well prepare for it."

In this last stage, individuals begin to come to terms with their mortality, or that of a loved one, or other tragic event. This stage varies according to the person's situation. People dying can enter this stage a long time before the people they leave behind, who must pass through their own individual stages of dealing with the grief.

---

**Bipolar Syndrome** is the patient's inability to control his mood swings and sometimes tends to have outbursts or depression. The patient presents with a passive aggressive nature. In some cases, patients may suffer from euphoria. Mood swings ranging from maniac behaviour to major depression is found in about 1% of normal human beings. This figure is far greater in Multiple Sclerosis than the norm. You will note that I refer to it as Bipolar Syndrome and not Bipolar itself. Bipolar Syndrome is more a manifestation of a symptom of MS and /or its medication than the actual disease Bipolar. Not much literature is available on the Syndrome, but small study groups show Bipolar like symptoms to be present in about 13% in MS patients. A leading contributing factor in corticosteroid treatment is sometimes mood swings.

Mood swings in Multiple Sclerosis are quite common as it is as wide spread as the symptoms of MS itself. Mood changes are directly correlated with the disease's effect on the person itself. Multiple Sclerosis symptoms vary in most cases from day to day, so too does your feeling of wellbeing or lack of it. Person with severe MS is more affected by this than those with Relapsing Remitting Multiple Sclerosis. However that being said, relapses play a major part in your feeling of wellbeing. Certain relapses can be very bad, and the patient will be in either in a severe depression, or an angry mood, but that is to be expected given the gravity of the disease itself.

The saddest after effect of this, is a very real phenomenon of Multiple Sclerosis. Now here is where I need to tread with caution, but it needs to be mentioned, so if I step on certain peoples toes here, so be it. In the vast majority of relationship failures, mood swings are used as an excuse by the partner to get out of the relationship, or marriage. Yes, in some cases mood swings are a very real factor affecting MS patients and their relationships, but it is also the biggest blaming tool or excuse as well. Living with a person with severe MS can be very difficult and only a very strong bond will survive it. I will elaborate on this a bit later on in the book.

Most symptoms of Bipolar Syndrome or mood swings can be controlled by medication.

# Treatments for Multiple Sclerosis

Before I get into the long list of treatments for Multiple Sclerosis I need to touch base with you with a little history in the treatment of MS from the past.

Probably the treatment of Multiple Sclerosis in the early 18th century to late in the 19th century was bloodletting. Bloodletting was a common practice for many diseases. This practice required the physician, or quacks to drain a certain percentage of the blood from the system. The reasoning behind this was that in getting rid of the so called bad blood, the body would heal. Luckily today in the 20th century we are spared this horrible experience. However with that being said, there are a small group of quacks mostly in Third World countries, that still believe in this.  A very Interesting rumour is that President George Washington had nearly 80 ounces of his blood drained in the final hours before his death, in the hope of curing him. Sadly it did not work and he passed away from Pneumonia a couple of hours later. The practice of bloodletting was advocated as late as 1942 in one of Sir William Osler's highly regarded medical textbooks. Sir William Osler a Canadian physician was one of the founding members of John's Hopkins hospital.

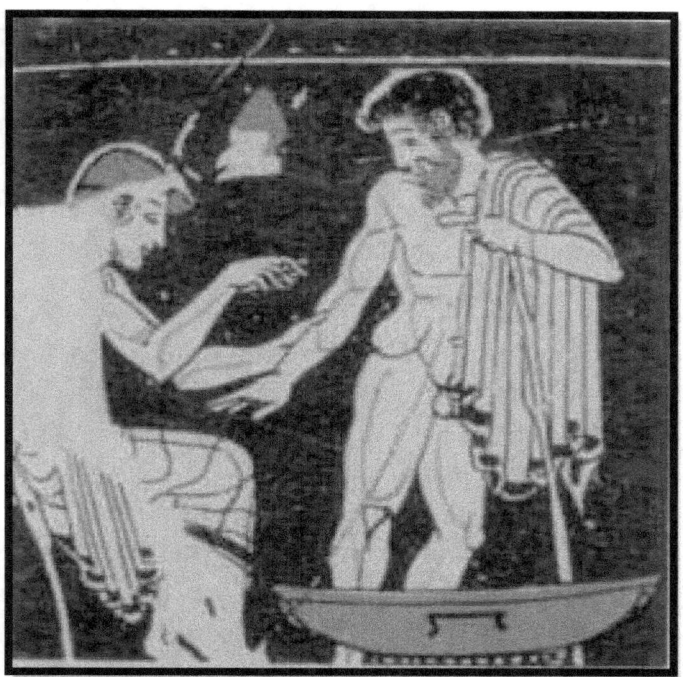

[53] The Ancient art of Bloodletting

In the 1890 it was believed that Multiple Sclerosis was caused by the suppression of sweat and was treated with herbs and bed rest. In 1910 the physicians believed that MS was caused by toxins in the blood and was treated by means of purging the patient and stimulants were given to the patient. By the year 1940 the thinking was that MS is caused by poor blood circulation and blood clots. These patients were treated with medicine to improve blood circulation.

In 1960 the doctors believed that Multiple Sclerosis was caused by some sort of allergic reaction and the patients were treated with vitamins and antihistamines. Modern diagnosis of Multiple Sclerosis was only in the late 1970. The ideas around MS had changed and steroids were used for the first time on MS patient. The early 1990s showed the introduction of the new MS Disease modifying drugs (DMD) medication as we know it today.

But let us not forget the famous Dr Freud who believed that MS or Creeping Paralysis was a state of the mind or female hysteria and the patient could be cured by talking to him. I am still of the opinion that this is why some Neurologists still believe that pain associated with MS is all in the mind and psychotherapy is needed to cure the patient. At least today modern medicine has evolved and we can treat Multiple Sclerosis with more effective drugs.

**Amitriptyline** is a Tricyclic anti-depressant with various names like Elavil, Enval, Endep and others. There are many of them on the market. Elavil is the most commonly describe in the United States and Canada

Now I know your first question is why an anti-depressant? To answer this, it is as effective as a painkiller as it recruits Delta Opioid Receptors (DOR) to combat pain. Opiate receptors are distributed widely in the brain, and are found in the spinal cord and digestive tract .This is your body's own pain mechanism. A lower dosage of Amitriptyline helps your body to recruit these "DOR". It is a so called off- label prescription as it was not designed to kill pain, but to help with depression. It has been found to be a very effective mechanism for neuropathic pain. Neuropathic pain is widely found in Multiple Sclerosis and is the direct result of damage to the sensory system of the brain. It is normally prescribed in a cocktail with either "Prozac" and or an anti-spasm medication like baclofen. The reason for this is achieve a mood stabilisation and help for spasms.

This medication may cause your skin to be more sensitive to sunlight than it is normally. Even brief exposure to sunlight may cause a skin rash, itching, redness or other discoloration of the skin, or severe sunburn. This medication may affect blood sugar levels of diabetic individuals. If you notice a change in the results of your blood or urine sugar tests, check with your physician.

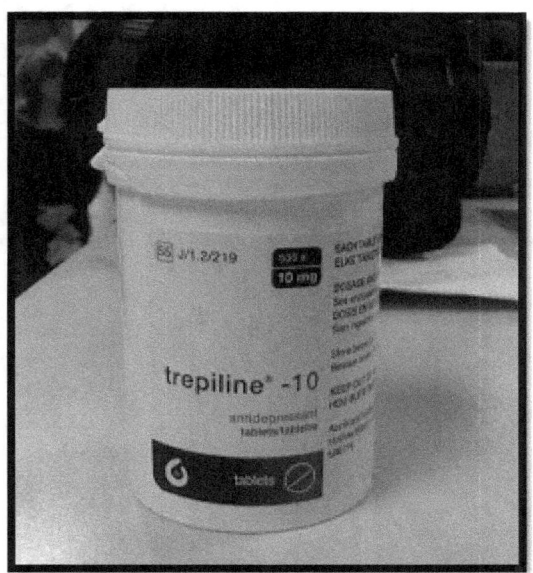

[54] Amitriptyline-Trepiline (Image courtesy of Flamwood Chemist)

Do not stop taking this medication without consulting your physician. The physician may want you to reduce the amount you are taking gradually in order to reduce the possibility of withdrawal symptoms such as headache, nausea, and/or an overall feeling of discomfort.

Side effects of amitriptyline are drowsiness, dry-mouth, and loss of appetite, sexual drive or weight gain. Other side effects include nervousness, constipation, blurred vision or dizziness. Rare side effects are tinnitus (ringing noise in ear), mania and psychosis. Irregular heart beat has been reported in rare cases.

**Carbamazepine** has a wide variety of market names which include the following Tegratol, Epitol, Calepsin, Treminol and Stazepine are just a few. It is an anticonvulsant that was first introduced in 1962 to treat Trigeminal Neuralgia or non-specific facial pain or neuropathic facial pain. It is also a mood stabilising drug. It is taken orally and the dosage varies in patients. Carbamazepine may also be used to treat Bipolar Syndrome in Multiple Sclerosis. The action of carbamazepine basically reduces the electric transmission in the brain and slows down the firing of electric energy between brain nerve endings.

Carbamazepine was discovered by chemist Walter Schindler at J.R. Geigy AG (now part of Novartis) in Basel, Switzerland, in 1953. Schindler then synthesized the drug in 1960, before its anti-epileptic properties had been discovered. It is what is called an off label treatment in Multiple Sclerosis, meaning it is used to treat , in this case Neuropathic pain, but it is not the drugs main intended treatment.

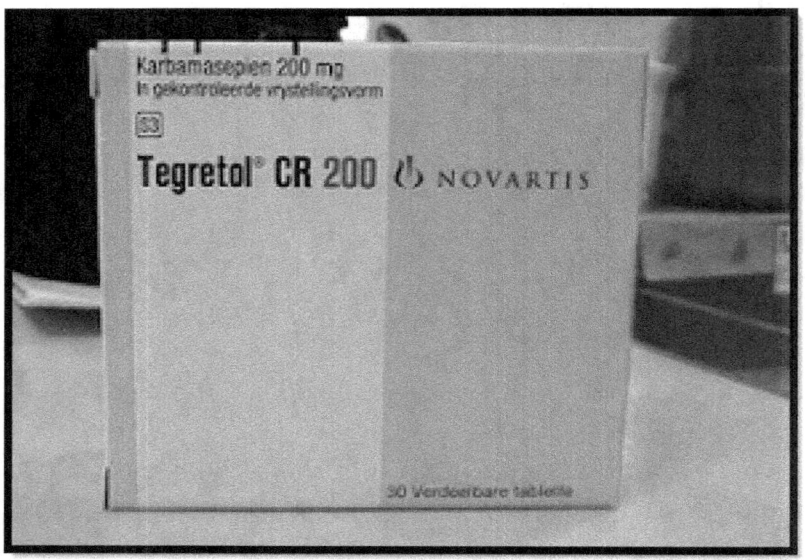

[55] Tegratol Tablets (Image courtesy of Flamwood Chemist)

Patients who use carbamazepine may become more sensitive to sunlight than they are normally used to. Exposure to sunlight, even for brief periods of time, may cause a skin rash, itching, redness of the skin, or severe sunburn and in cases visual sensitivity to sunlight.

Because of its wide ranging interaction with other drugs it should be given with extreme caution in conjunction with other drugs. It is one of the older drugs and is not used as often anymore. Side effects include drowsiness, headaches and co-ordination impairment. It may also cause stomach upset and greatly decreases a person's alcohol tolerance. Less common side effects are heart arrhythmia problems and blurred or double vision. In rare cases it causes a loss in the white blood cell count which may prove fatal, therefor you must have blood cell test when taken over a long period. Strange but true is it can also cause tone loss in the ears, where the tone a patient hears may drop a level or two. Carbamazepine is marketed by Novartis, but the patent rights have expired and a lot of generics are available.

**Gabapentin or Neurontin** is an anti-convulsant that is widely used for the treatment of neuropathic pain. The exact way gabapentin works is not known, but it seems to bind the calcium electron transmitters in the central nervous system. It is taken orally before bedtime as it leads to drowsiness.  It reduces pain and spasticity in Multiple sclerosis patients. It may also help to treat nystagmus or jerky movement in the eyes. It is also prescribe for MS patient suffering from restless leg syndrome. This drug has been on the market from 1994 but was first introduced for treatment of neuropathic pain in 2002. It is very similar to Pregabalin (Lyrica).

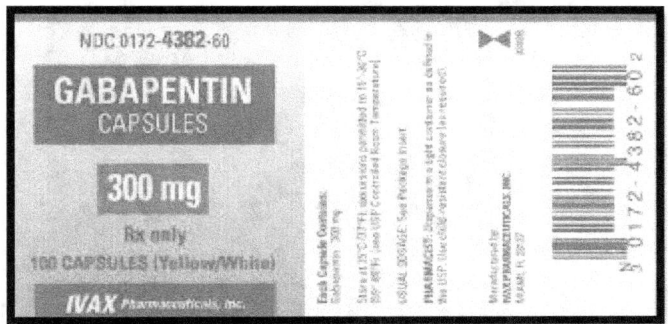

[56] Gabapentin or Neurontin (Image source National Library of Medicine (NLM))

Gabapentin's most common side effects are drowsiness, dizziness and swelling of the hands and feet. To suddenly discontinue using this medication may cause withdrawal symptoms. It should be given with care to patients that have kidney problems which could lead to toxic levels of the drug. Gabapentin has been associated with an increased risk of suicidal acts or violent deaths. The manufacturer has been taken to court in 2009 relating to the increase suicide risk.

Gabapentin is best known under the brand name Neurontin manufactured by Pfizer.

**Lyrica or Pregabalin** is an anti-convulsant that is prescribed for MS patients that suffer from neuropathic or non-specific pain disorders.  It is effective in the treatment of Trigeminal Neuralgia and optic neuritis and other neuropathic pain. It basically reduces the nervous system's transfer of electrical energy between the nerves by suppressing the calcium uptake of the nervous system. It is also prescribed for panic disorders. Patients are not as prone to became addicted to it, than on the older drugs. The drug has been on the market since 2004.

Lyrica may cause serious, even life threatening, allergic reactions. Once you stop taking Lyrica, see your doctor immediately if you have any signs of a serious allergic reaction. Some signs are swelling of your face, mouth, lips, gums, tongue, throat or neck or if you have any trouble breathing, or have a rash, hives or blisters. It is associated with suicidal tendencies in a very small number of people, about 1 in 500.

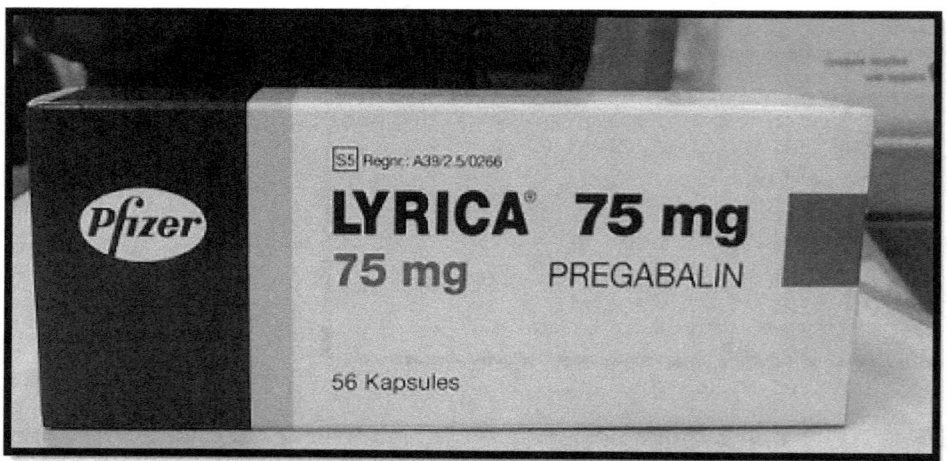

[57] Lyrica Tablets(Image courtesy of Flamwood Chemist)

The main side effect is drowsiness and dizziness. Common side effects are blurred vision, tremors, memory loss and euphoria. It can also cause weight gain and decrease of your libido. Constipation and a dry mouth are also side effects. Less frequent side effects include depression, confusion and agitation. Some patients also suffer from hallucinations. Very rare side effects include a low white blood cell that could lead to infections. Other side effects include heart or blood flow problems, although this is extremely rare.

Pregabalin was invented by medicinal chemist Richard Bruce Silverman at North-western University in the United States. Lyrica or pregabalin is marketed by Pfizer.

**Azathioprine** or Imuran, Imurel or Azumun is an anti-rejection drug and immune suppressant. It is primarily designed for organ transplants but is also used to treat autoimmune disease like Multiple Sclerosis and Rheumatoid Arthritis. It has been on the market for a long time and is one of the older immune suppressants used to treat Multiple Sclerosis. The medication is taken as an oral dosage and is an older generation of drugs used to treat Progressive Multiple Sclerosis.

The side effects of this drug are hair loss, nausea and fatigue. Another complication of this drug is bone marrow suppression that leads to opportunistic infections. Drug toxicity is also common and you need regular blood work to check toxicity levels. It is also not indicated in pregnancy or during breast feeding.

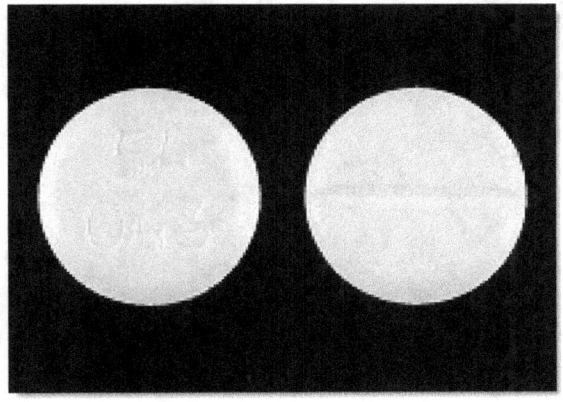

[58] Azathioprine (Image source National Library of Medicine (NLM))

As this is an older drug on the market and it is hardly used to treat Multiple Sclerosis anymore. In Neuromyelitis Optica it is still used as a treatment with corticosteroids, and in some Third World countries as a main treatment for Multiple Sclerosis, due to economic constraints.

**Baclofen** (Kemstro, Lioresal, Liofen, Gablofen, and Beklo) is anti-spasm medication. It works by blocking the sodium channels in the nerves from opening. So when the potential firing action of the neurotransmitters stops firing, it halts spasms from occurring. In other words, it stops the electrical transmissions in cell endings in the nerves. Baclofen was originally designed for epilepsy patients in 1920, but the results were not as expected. Why it was introduced to treat for spasticity in spinal injuries is unknown. It is also helpful in the treatment of trigeminal neuralgia. In 2012 Baclofen was approved to be used to treat alcohol addiction in alcoholics. One doctor used it to treat his own alcohol addiction.

Muscles receive electrical impulses via nerves to contract and relax. Spasticity is caused by an imbalance of electrical impulses coming from the spinal cord through the nerves to the muscle. This imbalance causes the muscle to become hyperactive, resulting in involuntary spasms. Baclofen works by restoring the normal balance and reducing muscle hyperactivity. In this way, it allows for more normal muscle movements.

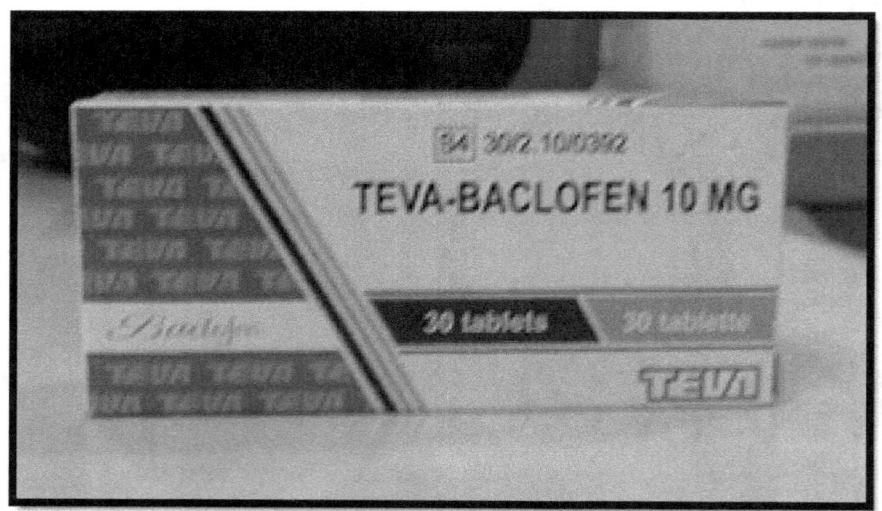

[59] Baclofen Tablets (Image courtesy of Flamwood Chemist)

This also used to treat muscle cramps, stiffness and for the treatment of pain in MS. It can be taken orally or by means of a pump implanted in the patient. In about 5% of MS patients baclofen does not seems to help. The dosage from patient to patient varies, from 10mg upwards. If the meds are suddenly stopped withdrawal symptoms may appear. Normal side effects like drowsiness are common in baclofen. It may also lead to a slow reaction time and impair your thinking. So be careful when driving or using machinery. Other side effects include dizziness, headaches, nausea and weakness.

Baclofen is taken orally but can be given by means of an intrathecal baclofen pump system. The system consists of a catheter and a pump. The pump, a round metal disc, about one inch thick and three inches in diameter, is surgically placed under the skin of the abdomen near the waistline. This way doctors can deliver baclofen directly into the spinal fluid.

The pump releases the prescribed amounts of medicine through the catheter which is programmable by an eternal programmer. The external programmer can make adjustments to the dosage, rate, and timing of the medication. The pump is only refillable in a Doctor's office and is replaced after the battery lifespan is reached in 5-7 years. New studies indicate that tolerance may develop in some patients receiving intrathecal baclofen treatment.

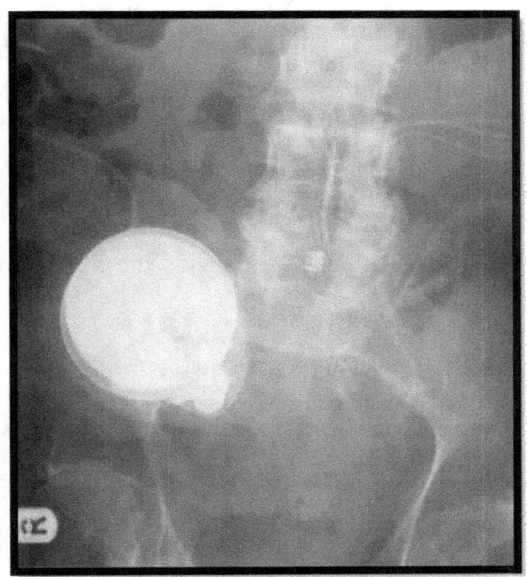

[60] Baclofen Pump x-ray Image (Source: National Library of Medicine (NLM))

**Ampyra or Fampridine** is marketed under the name Ampyra or dalfampridine. It is not a DMD as such on its own, but rather an assisted drug to the DMD to reduce the symptoms. Ampyra is normally prescribed to patients with any type of MS to improve muscle strength, and is listed as safe to use with Disease Modifying Drugs.

A successful phase II trial was completed in 2008 named the MS-F204 trial, including 204 patients and control groups. They then went onto phase III trials in 2009. Phase III trials consisted of 301 patients and a control group. It received the FDA approval for release of this drug in the market, on 22 Jan 2010. Fampridine is a selective potassium calcium blocker. Basically it interferes with the production of potassium that causes an increase in iron deposits; in turn this reduces the damage created by increased potassium which is damaging to Myelin. It reduces the amount of potassium which in turn reduces the duration and strength of iron deposits on the Myelin thus reducing the damaging effects. A reduce dosage benefits the burden of treatment to the patients.

The biggest result that has come from the clinical trial showed it to improve the debilitating effects in walking speed and muscle strength. However, it will not repair the permanent damage that has already been done by the Demyelination process. It is mostly intended for patients who still have progression in their MS symptoms, and can still be helped by this medication. The results also show a reduction in the amount of lesions on the brain (Still to be verified). It has shown to have a fourfold effect on a Multiple Sclerosis patient. It is indicated for patients who have muscle weakness and difficulty walking with multiple Sclerosis.

1. It decreases the rate of relapses. (Still to be verified)

2. It prevents disability directly associated with a relapse. (Increases the ability to walk)

3. It provides management of symptoms directly related to fixed neurological deficits which include walking ability and speed.

4. It prevents direct disability arising directly from the disease's progression in the strengthening of the legs.

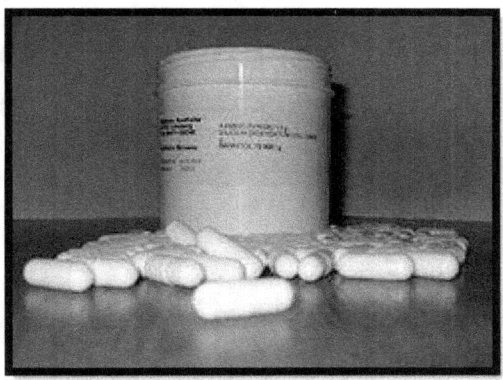

[61] Ampyra or Fampridine (Image source: Wikipedia. Author:    Radosław Drożdżewski)

The main advantage of this drug is that it improves the muscles' strength and increases the ability to walk. This drug is taken on a daily oral dosage. Some side effects should be noted. It is not recommended for patients that have seizures or kidney dysfunction. Patients should mention this to their doctors before taking this drug. The dosage is 10mg twice daily, higher dosages can cause seizure.  Side effects are nausea, dizziness, urinary tract infections, balance disorder, swelling of nose and throat. Also reported is diarrhoea and constipation. But as with any meds, we can expect side effects and these side effects present in about only 5% of patients. Ampyra is marketed Acorda Therapeutics

**Provigil or Modafinil** is given to Multiple Sclerosis patient to treat the symptoms of brain fatigue. This drug increases the brain dopamine and other brain norepinephrine hormones in the brain. This leads to an increase in the hormones that increases the brains' wakefulness. In other words, it increases the neurotransmitters in the brain that lead to fatigue. It is used as an off label treatment to treat the symptoms of severe fatigue in Multiple Sclerosis patients. It also increases the working ability of the brain and the digit span of the patient. It may also be helpful to increase the cognitive function of the brain to a certain extent. It also helps to increase the brain's pattern memory. It is mostly given to Multiple Sclerosis patients to alter the brains wakefulness and decrease the level of fatigue. This drug helps to decrease mental and physical fatigue.

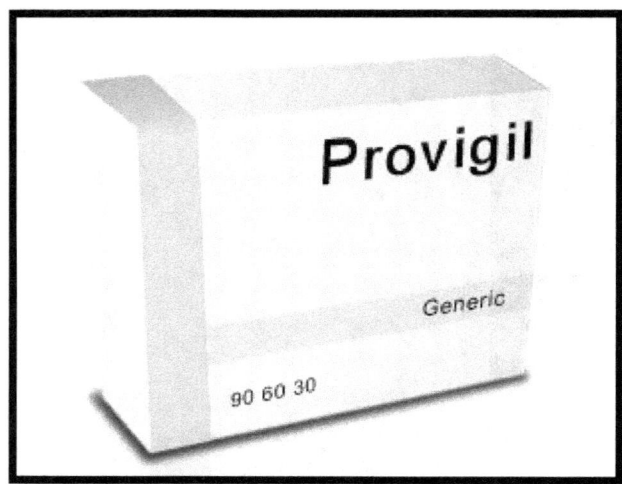

[62] Provigil

The prescribed label dosage is normally for a maintenance dosage over time or else it is taken by the patient on self-noticed fatigue days.

Common side effects are sleep disorders, anxiety, nervousness, aggressiveness, irritability, and confusion. Also reported is nausea and diarrhoea. It can lead to excitement or agitation in some patients. Extreme care should be used in patients with a history of heart problems. Adverse side effects are that, it can lead to Dress Syndrome or Stephan Johnsen syndrome, which are both drug reaction syndromes and can in rare cases, be fatal.

Modafinil was originally developed in France by neurophysiologist and emeritus experimental medicine professor Michel Jouvet and Lafon Laboratories in the late 1970. It is marketed by Cephalon, Inc., a wholly-owned subsidiary of Teva Pharmaceutical. The patent right has lapsed and it now available as a generic as well with names like Alertec, Carim, Modalert, Modasomil, Modavigil, Modiodal, Provigil, Resotyl, Stavigile, Vigia, Vigicer and Vigil.

**Sativex spray** is used to treat pain in cancer patient in clinical trials. Sativex has also shown to help with neuropathic pain and spasticity in Multiple Sclerosis. Sativex also relieves over-active bladder problems. Sativex is used as mouth spray, under the tongue or the inner cheeks. It is proving to be very positive for relieve of pain and spasticity. It has also been tested for sleep disorders and show signs of improvement of sleep patterns.

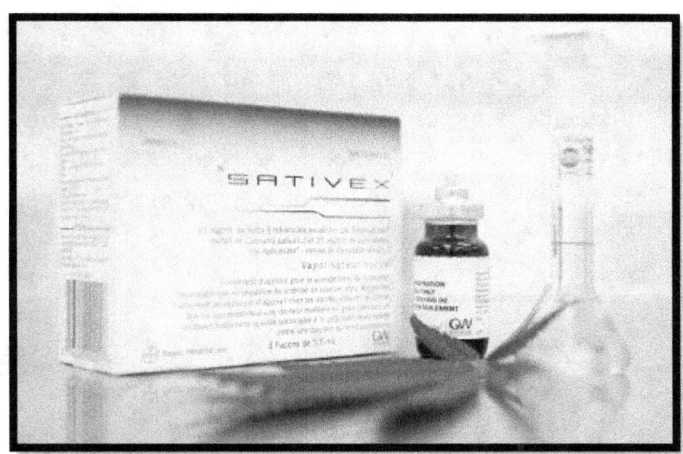

[63] Sativex Spray (Picture Courtesy of GW Pharmaceuticals plc.)

The main compound of Sativex is Tetrahydrocannibol and Cannibidiol. The abbreviations are TCH and CBD. It is manufactured from the cannabis plant or for those who don't know, "Marijuana". It is a medical Marijuana extract. It is currently the only genuine extract of TCH and OCB; all other products with TCH are manufactured synthetically. It was approved for use in the Canada in 2005 under strict control. Currently there is a large trial for this medication and this will be completed in 2013, although these studies are mostly for pain in cancer patients. In Catalonia, Spain it was tested on about 600 patients with MS. It is not legal in most countries. It is controlled very strictly, as cannabis is an illegal drug, in the majority of countries. Sativex has been developed as a result of patients smoking cannabis for pain, thus removing the illegal risk component. However legalisation is still complicated in many countries.

The spray is tolerated quite well by patients and there are very little side effects. Most common side effects are dizziness, dry mouth, drowsiness and nausea. Some respiratory tract infections have also been reported. Patient that do stop taking Sativex show little or no withdrawal symptoms. Some patients have reported no or little relief with Sativex.

Sativex spray is marketed by GW Pharmaceuticals plc.

**Botox** has been an off label treatment for a couple of years to relieve spasticity in Multiple Sclerosis. This Allergan received approval from the FDA to use Botox for treatment in the upper limbs for spasticity in multiple sclerosis. Botox has had three very successful studies in relieving upper limb spasticity in Multiple Sclerosis. The study's aim was to relieve spastic hands, elbows and shoulders in Multiple Sclerosis patients. This is relatively common in MS, affecting the patient's movement of the arms, hands and shoulders. Botox is also injected into the bladder muscle in MS patients to relieve the embarrassing symptom of a leaky bladder.

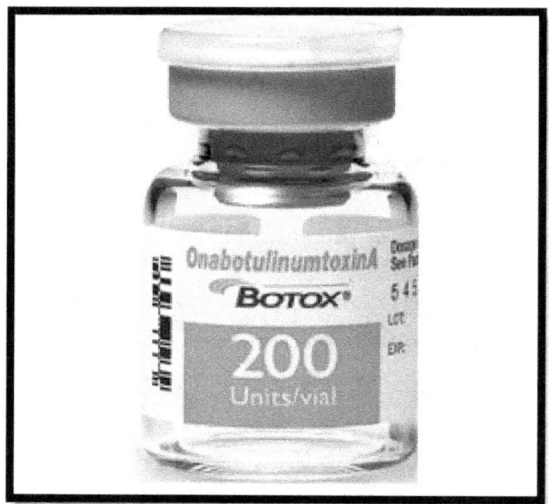

[64] Botox

Botox is a Botulinum toxin, a neurotoxic protein produced by the bacterium called clostridium Botulinum. It is used in very small dosages that are injected into the affected muscle, thus causing the reduction in muscle activity, thus reducing the spasms. This action is derived when Botox blocks the neurotransmitters to the muscles. It is used also used in neck stiffness and can help for eye muscle jerking as well.

The side effects off Botox are minimal and normally disappear quickly after the injection. The most common side effect is a stinging sensation and bruising at the injection site. However serious allergic reactions have been reported. These reactions include itching, rash, red itchy welts, wheezing, asthma symptoms, or dizziness or feeling faint.

Botox is not new to the market as it has been used from 1980 onwards for cosmetic reasons

# Disease Modifying Drugs (DMD)

Disease modifying drugs consist of mostly Interferons. Interferons bind to neighbouring cells and stimulate these cells to produce antiviral proteins which can prevent viral replication in these cells. The name interferon stems from their ability to "interfere" with viral replication within host cells. Interferons are a family of naturally occurring proteins in the human body that are made and secreted by cells of the immune system. For example, white blood cells, natural killer cells, fibroblasts, and epithelial cells. There are three Classes of Interferon's:

1.  Alpha,

2.  Beta

3.  Gamma.

The Beta class is used in Multiple Sclerosis. Interferon beta-1b and interferon beta-1a are approved for the treatment of Multiple Sclerosis. The other two classes are used to treat cancer and other diseases. Each class has many effects, though their effects overlap. Commercially available interferons are human interferons' manufactured using DNA technology. The way it works is complex and to avoid confusion I will not dwell on it, only on the fact that it does work by reducing relapses.

**Avonex** is an Interferon beta-1a and provides the lowest dosage per week. The way AVONEX works to fight the disease is not known but to understand how AVONEX is thought to work, it helps to know more about how MS affects your brain. The Cerebral Spinal Fluid in your brain is protected from substances in your blood by a wall of cells known as the blood-brain barrier. This barrier protects the brain from blood or T-killer blood cells and helper B cells from entering the brain. In patients who have MS, holes appear in your Blood Brain Barrier which allows immune cells to cross into your Cerebral Spinal Fluid (CSF) where they can cause damaging inflammation or lesions. Avonex has been available since 1995. It is made by Biogen Idec.

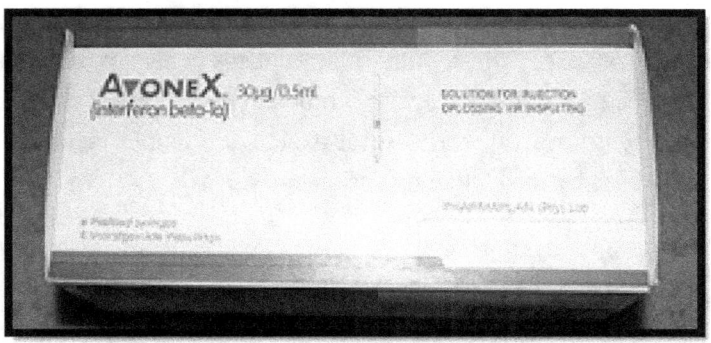

[65] Avonex (Image courtesy of Tanya Piper)

Avonex works by reducing the gaps or holes in the Blood Brain Barrier as well as to modify immune cells outside your CNS. If these modified cells cross the blood-brain barrier, they will work to fight MS inflammation instead of causing it. Study's has shown it decreases relapses to as much as 32%   in RRMS.

Avonex is delivered by an injection once a week intramuscular (normally the thigh area) and a new dosage pen is now available making the experience more comfortable. AVONEX PEN is a single-use prefilled auto injector that uses a covered needle that's half the length of the standard needle for AVONEX Prefilled Syringe.

The side effects of Avonex are similar to those of other interferon-based therapies; however Avonex does not cause as many injection-site reactions as the others. You may experience flu-like symptoms, liver problems, decreased blood counts, injection site itch or rash, and depression. Severe symptoms reported are heart problems, seizures and low bone marrow platelet counts

Avonex should be used with caution in patients with depression, as it can cause hallucination and suicidal thoughts.

**Betaseron** also an Interferon, but a beta-1b has been on the market longer than any other disease-modifying drugs. It provides the highest weekly dose of all interferon's, at 250mcg/dose, given every other day. It is a subcutaneous or in other words under the skin formula and has a neutral pH, as opposed to Avonex which is injected into the muscle. It defers from Rebif which is also a subcutaneous injection, but Rebif is acidic, so injections can be painful.

Betaseron will not cure your MS but may help decrease how often you experience multiple sclerosis flare-ups or relapses. The reduction in relapses is also about 33% as with Avonex. Due to the higher dosage, certain studies indicate fewer relapse than Avonex or Rebif. The way Betaseron works is not exactly known. Betaseron is thought to reduce RRMS relapses by the following actions:

1. Blocking certain immune system cells—called T cells—from attacking Myelin, the material that protects your nerve axons

2. Stopping certain types of proteins from activating the immune system to attack your Myelin

3. Reducing the gaps in the blood brain barrier.

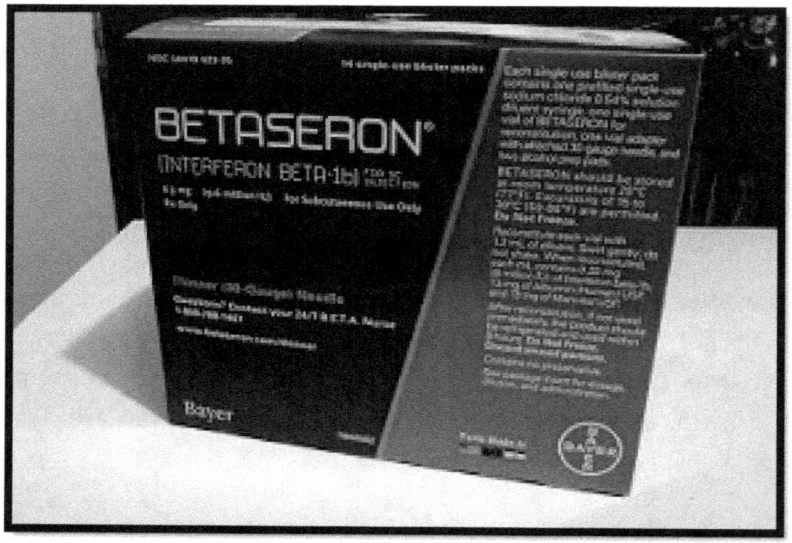

[66] Betaseron (Image courtesy of Laura Weber)

Usual interferon-related, flu-like symptoms, especially at the beginning of treatment accompany Betaseron treatment. However, Betaseron begins with a titration schedule, meaning patients start with a small dose and increase it gradually. This is done to greatly reduce the side effects. Betaseron requires mixing and can be stored at room temperature, making it convenient for travel. Patients do require blood tests performed regularly to monitor liver function and white blood cell count. Betaseron also comes with an auto injector called Betaject 3.

The side effects of Betaseron are very similar to Avonex. Betaseron trade names include Betaferon, Betaseron (North America), Extavia and Ziferon. Betaseron was introduced into the market by Bayer HealthCare and is the longest on the market, since 1993. Novartis has also introduced Extavia, a new brand of interferon beta-1b, in 2009.

**Rebif** is basically the same formulation as Avonex and also Interferon beta-1a. Rebif has a higher dosage than Avonex. Rebif has been shown to be slightly more effective than Avonex at preventing relapses and can be attributed to its higher dosage and is given three times a week. Patients do experience more injection site reactions, more liver disorders and white blood cell disorders. However, a patient tends to experience less flu-like symptoms over time, and they seem to last for a shorter period after dosing. Rebif is injected subcutaneously or in plain English, under the skin. It does have the smallest needle on the market.

Rebif has a similar action to other interferons and the reduction in relapse is again placed at 33%.  It interferes with the immune systems cell reproduction and reduces the gaps in the endothelial cell layer of the blood brain vessel, effectively repairing the blood brain barrier to certain extent. It also reduces the inflammation process in the brains nerve axons.

Rebif is however acidic and more injection site reactions are noted, in the form of red spots or small swelling, with a stinging sensation at the injection area. This occurs at the site of injections in 71% of patients) which may last for weeks. They can break down into sores or so-called injection-site necrosis in 5% of all cases.

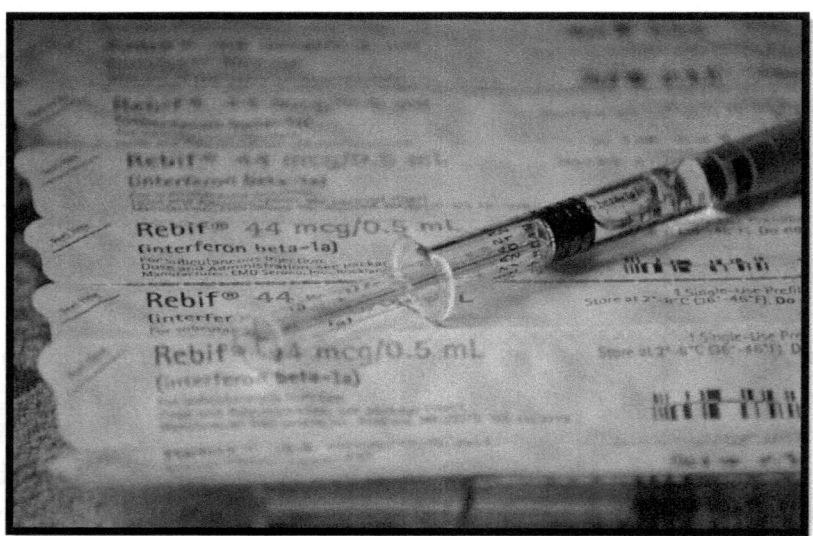

[67] Rebif prefilled syringes (Image courtesy of Michelle Baldwin)

Rebif as with any Interferons will not cure Multiple Sclerosis but it has been shown to decrease the number of flare-ups and slow the occurrence of some of the physical disability that is common in people with MS. Rebif is marketed by Merck Serono and Pfizer.

**Copaxone**, glatiramer acetate has a different formulation than the other CRAB drugs, which are interferon-based. Glatiramer acetate is an immune modulator drug currently used to treat Multiple Sclerosis. It is a random polymer of four amino acids found in myelin basic protein, namely glutamic acid, lysine, alanine, and tyrosine, and may work as a decoy for the immune system. Due to its resemblance to myelin basic protein, it acts as a sort of decoy, diverting an autoimmune response against Myelin. However it has no effect on the integrity of the blood brain barrier, at least not in the early stages of treatment. It has different side effects, which does not include flu-like symptoms, links to depression, potential liver damage or effects on white blood cells or thyroid function as in the case with interferons. This makes Copaxone a popular choice for people working full-time, mothers of young children or other people who cannot afford down time due to side effects.

Copaxone is injected daily, making it the most frequently used of any MS disease modifying drugs. It is also injected subcutaneously. Injection side effects include fairly itchy or painful welts that can take up to 5 days to heal. This is the most common side effect. Copaxone also can cause lipoatrophy, a destruction of fat cells in localized areas where it has been injected. This looks like a depression in the skin and underlying tissues and is permanent. Another side effect is acute panic attacks. Although it is normally short lived, about 10-15 minutes from the injection, it can be very scary. These reactions involve flushing, chest pain, heart palpitations, anxiety, constriction of the throat and/or trouble breathing.

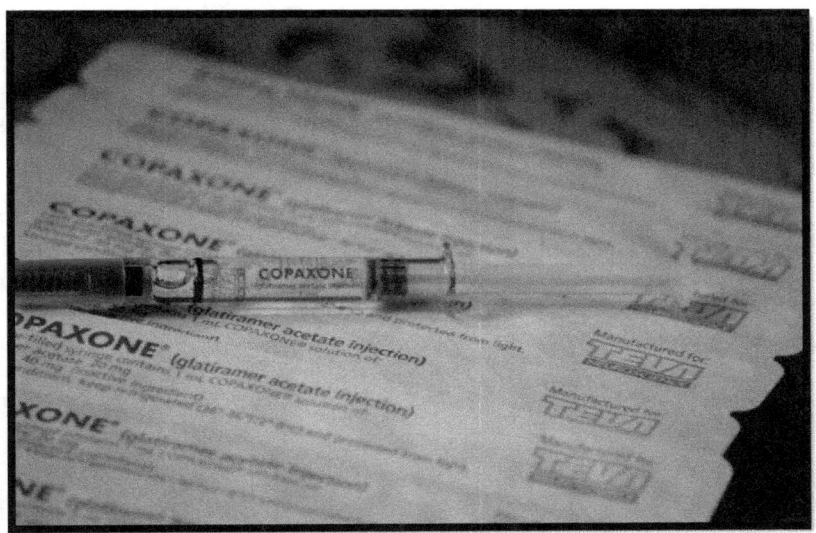

[68] Copaxone (Image courtesy of Michelle Baldwin)

The success rate of Copaxone is about 29% in the short term, but long term studies have indicated a reduction of 80% in relapses over ten years. In other words, they went from having 1.5 relapses per year to one relapse every 5 years.

Since Copaxone takes up to six month to reach its full potential, Neurologists are reluctant to start patients with more aggressive MS. Copaxone comes in prefilled syringes and no mixing or assembly is required before the injection time. They should be allowed to come to room temperature before injecting. Copaxone has been available since 1996 and is marketed as Copolymer 1, Cop-1, or Copaxone - as marketed by Teva Pharmaceuticals.

The four Disease Modifying Drugs are the mainline DMD and known as CRAB. There are some new disease modifying drugs out there and I will go through them.

**Tysabri** or **Natalizumab** has been developed for patients that do not tolerate or react to other MS Disease Modifying drugs. It is administered by means of a 300mg IV infusion every 28 days. The main effect of Tysabri is that it slows down the debilitating effects of Multiple Sclerosis, especially in slowing down vision loss. It is recommended for highly active Relapsing Remitting Multiple Sclerosis. The drug reduces the ability of inflammatory immune cells of crossing the blood brain barrier. It can also improve your quality of life drastically.

The symptom-causing lesions of MS are believed to be caused when inflammatory cells such as T-Killer cells pass through the blood brain barrier through the endothelial cells layer. Tysabri appears to reduce the transmission of immune cells into the Cerebral Fluid by interfering with molecules on the surfaces of these cells. Tysabri treatment led to a 68 % relative reduction in the annual relapse rate when compared with placebo and reduced the relative risk of disability progression by 42-54 %.

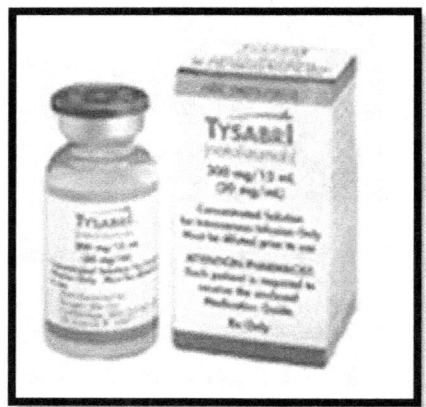

[69] Tysabri or Natalizumab (Image courtesy of anonymous patient)

However Tysabri has some side effects and has not been on the market for long. It has only been approved in 2004 and therefor there are no long term studies on this drug. The most common side effect is fatigue and allergic reaction. Headache and nausea and colds are also side effects but not as common, as well as allergic shock.

Tysabri can cause liver damage in rare cases. It is also not recommended for patients that have a weakened immune system as it may cause patients to develop a brain disease called progressive multifocal leukoencephalopathy or PML for short.

Tysabri comes with a big warning though after being recalled for a brief period from the market in 2005. PML or Progressive Multifocal Leukoencephalopathy is a very rare brain disease that can be fatal. It is a viral infection of the brain caused by the JC virus (first recorded in 1971), the initials of the first person from whom tissue sample it was cultivated. It is not a new disease; 70 - 90% of the population do have anti bodies in their blood, so the virus is quite widespread. Most of the world population has a latent form of this disease. All indication is that we are infected in our younger years with the JC virus.

When the immune system is severely suppressed it can cause the onset of this disease and as soon as the virus crosses the blood brain barrier it causes PML. PML is similar to Multiple Sclerosis but far more destructive than MS.

Tysabri is used to treat MS patients, when all of the other disease modifying drugs have not helped. It can suppress the immune system in such a matter, that it can cause the onset of PML. Strict control is being used in in patients on Tysabri to be aware of the early onset of PML. In its early stages it can still be treated with antiretroviral to stop the progress of PML (unconfirmed). But this is not purely associated with Tysabri. In some cases of Steroid treatment, especially in aggressive steroid use it can also lead to the onset of PML. PML is also noted in Aids patients, with 5% of these patients developing PML. Some cancer treatments can also cause PML.

In January, 2012, the FDA changed the labelling for Tysabri to indicate that the testing positive of JC virus antibodies has been shown to be a risk factor for PML. The FDA also approved the Stratify JCV Antibody ELISA test; a positive result on this test means that a person has been exposed to JCV in the past. Only Patients who have been exposed to JCV appear to be at risk of PML. The risks and benefits of starting or continuing treatment with Tysabri should be considered carefully in any person who is anti-JCV antibody positive and has one or more of the other known risk factors for PML. Regular blood testing is required.

There are other known risks factors including:

Longer time on treatment with Tysabri – especially over two years

Prior treatment with an immunosuppressant medication (e.g., mitoxantrone, azathioprine, methotrexate, cyclophosphamide, or mycophenolate mofetil)

A person who tests positive for anti-JCV antibodies but has no other risk factors has a less than 1 in 1000 risk of developing PML. A person with all three risk factors has an 11 in 1000 risk of developing PML. It is co-marketed by Biogen Idec and Élan as Tysabri, and was previously named Antegren.

On August 15, 2012, the FDA required another change to the prescribing information, recommending that patients with a negative anti-JCV antibody test result should be retested every 6 months. The known cases of PML developing in Tysabri treatments are 302 patients since its introduction in 2006.

The good news is that certain treatments can possibly cure PML. All these are still in trial but look promising and are being done to create a safe platform for Tysabri. So some MS Specialists are rather waiting for the outcome of a safer platform before prescribing this drug. The new suggestion is that patients should take drug holidays to give the body's immune system time to repair it and reduce the chances of developing PML.

When you are being treated with Tysabri you should take great care in noticing any changes in your symptoms. The symptoms of PML and MS are closely related. Inform your neurologist if you should have any symptoms of, or related to both that has worsened as it may be a sign of PML. If caught early enough PML can still be reversed.

**Gilenya** (Fingolimod or FTY720) is an oral immune Suppressant that was designed for kidney transplant patient originally. It works by suppressing the white blood cells, Killer T-Cells or B-Helper cells in the body. In short, it reduces the amount of antibodies in the blood, by reducing the manufacture of white blood cells that carry Killer T-Cells and helper B-Cells. It produces a condition that is called Lymphocytopenia, a condition that is associated with a low white blood cell count. Gilenya does not cure MS, but like interferons, it slows down relapses. Gilenya reduces the number of relapses by 52% compared to interferons. Patients that remained 1 year relapse free were 83% compared 72% of those on interferons.

After 2 years, people taking GILENYA were 30% less likely to have physical disability progression.

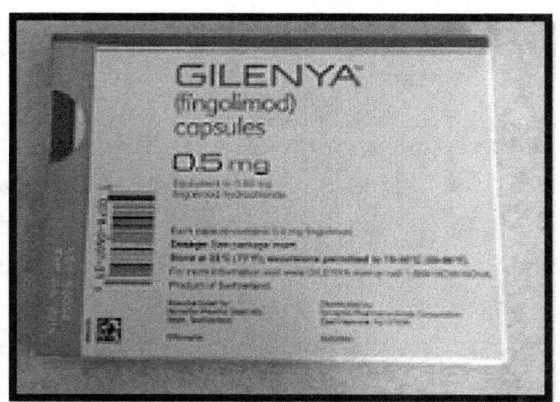

[70] Gilenya Tablets (Image courtesy of Kelly O'Donnell)

First synthesized in 1992, Fingolimod was derived from Myriocin which possesses immunosuppressant activity. Myriocin was isolated from the culture broth a type of entomopathogenic fungus the "Isaria sinclairii" that was an eternal youth nostrum in traditional Chinese medicine. Showing positive results in prolonging rat skin graft survival time, myriocin was modified through a series of steps to form Fingolimod, named at the time FTY720.

It has now completed the Freedom trials or phase III trials, a double blind study in Relapsing Remitting Multiple Sclerosis. The results were a drop in relapse per year 0.18 compared to 0.4 in the placebo control group. This result was with the 0.5mg per day dosage. In the other control study where the dosage was 1.25mg per day the results were similar. The relapse rate in this group was 0.16 per year as compared to the 0.4 in the control group. The disease follow up test in two years has shown a 0.7 and 0.68 drop in progression compared to the control group. The resulting MRI studies also reported better result on the Gilenya group compared to the placebo group. The number of lesions was estimated to be about 50% less than the placebo group and also statistically to the amount of lesions expected over a two year period.

Certain adverse side effects have caused that certain patients were removed from the clinical trials. The majority of the serious side effects were reported in the larger dosage group. Heart beat irregularities was reported in certain cases in the initial dosage. Respiratory tract infections including bronchitis and pneumonia were reported. In the high dosage control group this was 9.6% compared to the 6% in the lower dosage. The most common side effects in the clinical trials of Gilenya were headache, influenza, diarrhoea, back pain, abnormal liver tests, and cough.

It went into public advisory subcommittee hearings on the 10 June 2010 and was given the green light for approval. In 2011 on September, 22 it was approved as a treatment for Multiple Sclerosis in the USA, and soon after that in Canada and Europe. It is marketed under the name Gilenya and the dosage regime will be 0,5Mg orally per day. This was the largest trial ever submitted to the FDA with over 7 years of studies and 4500 participants. To date this drug has been proven to be the most effective drug to treat MS compared to interferons.

You need a couple of tests before you can use it and they are as follows.

1.  A new or recent blood test to establish lymphocyte (immune cell) count

2.  An eye (ophthalmologic) evaluation; Gilenya can cause a swelling of the macula, a spot in the centre of retina of the eye, generally within 3-4 months of starting treatment. Macular Edema can cause symptoms similar to those that occur with an attack of optic neuritis, or may not be noticed at all. It is recommended that your doctor test your vision before starting treatment and then three to four months later, or any time that you notice any changes in your vision, including blurriness or shadows in the centre of your vision, a blind spot in the centre of your vision, sensitivity to light, or changes in your colour vision.

3.  A new or recent blood test to evaluate liver enzyme levels;

4.  A new or recent electrocardiogram in those using heart medications, those who have cardiac risk factors, or those who on examination have slow or irregular heart beat prior to starting Gilenya

5.  Those that do not have a history of chickenpox or vaccination against varicella zoster virus (VZV) should be tested for VZV antibodies, and those who are negative should consider vaccination before starting treatment with Gilenya.

Gilenya can result in a slow heart rate when first taken. Your first dose will be given in a medical facility where you will be watched for at least 6 hours. If you stop taking Gilenya for more than 14 days after your first month of treatment, you will need to repeat this observation. Gilenya (Fingolimod) is marketed by Novartis and is the first oral disease modifying drug on the market.

**AUBAGIO (teriflunomide)** is a prescription medicine used to treat relapsing forms of Multiple Sclerosis. AUBAGIO can decrease the number of Multiple Sclerosis flare-ups. AUBAGIO can help slow down the physical problems that MS causes but it is not a cure for MS. It is the second oral disease modifying drug approved for use in Multiple Sclerosis.

Teriflunomide is an immune system modulating drug reducing rapidly dividing cells, including killer T and B immune cells that are active in MS and also inhibits the production of immune messenger chemicals by T cells in Multiple Sclerosis. Teriflunomide may decrease the risk of infections compared to chemotherapy drugs used in Multiple Sclerosis because of its more-limited effects on the immune system.

In the TEMSO Phase III trial involving 1088 people with relapsing MS of which 796 completed the trial, oral Aubagio reduced relapses compared with the placebo over at least 108 weeks. Two different doses tested during the TEMSO including a 7 mg and 14 mg dose. The higher dose slowed progression of disability in patients. Both doses also had a favourable effect on several MRI tests. The results included a smaller increase in total lesion volume and fewer new and active lesions compared with the placebo.

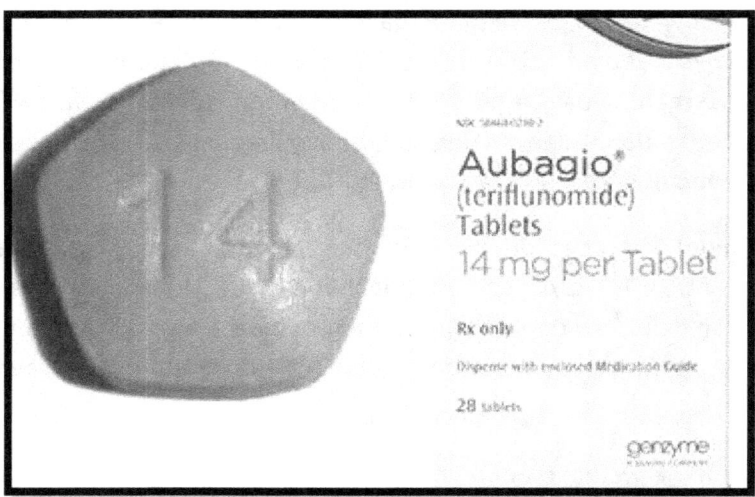

[71] Aubagio

Aubagio (7mg or 14mg) is a tablet taken once per day by mouth, with or without food.

Before you start using this medication, your doctor should do the following tests:

- A new or recent (within six months) blood test to detect levels of liver enzymes and a Complete Blood Count (CBC) to determine levels of blood cells.

- Blood pressure check

- Screening test for tuberculosis

- A pregnancy test in women

Aubagio should not be used in pregnant women, and you and your partner should be using birth control before using this medication. AUBAGIO may stay in your blood for up to 2 years after you stop taking it. Your doctor can prescribe a medicine that can help remove AUBAGIO from your body quicker.

Before you start AUBAGIO, tell your doctor if you have: liver or kidney problems; a fever or infection; numbness or tingling in your hands or feet; diabetes, serious skin problems when taking other medications; breathing problems; high blood pressure; or if you are breast feeding or plan to breast feed.

The most common side effects of AUBAGIO include:

- Abnormal liver test results

- Hair thinning

- Diarrhoea

- Flu

- Nausea

- A burning or prickling feeling in your skin.

Aubagio is marketed in the U.S. and in Australia.  Aubagio is marketed by the drug company Genzyme.

**Tecfidera (BG-12)** passed a successful Phase III clinical development trial for the treatment of Relapsing-Remitting Multiple Sclerosis (RRMS), the most common form of Multiple Sclerosis, and has been approved by the FDA.  The medical use of fumaric acid was first described in 1959 by the German chemist W. Schweckendiek and is not new to the market.

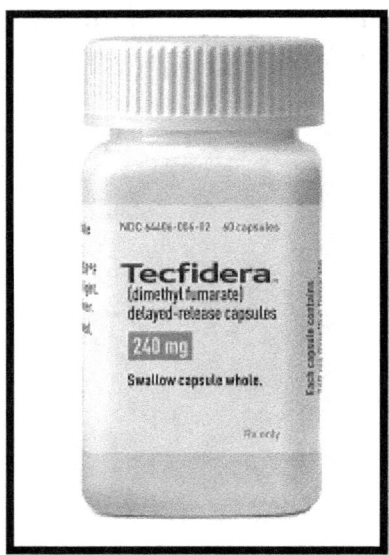

[72] Tecfidera - BG 12

Dimethyl fumarate is a form of fumaric acid. In patients with Relapsing-Remitting Multiple Sclerosis, dimethyl fumarate (BG-12) significantly reduced relapses and disability progression in a phase 3 trial. It activates the Nrf2 antioxidant response pathway, the primary cellular defence against the cytotoxic effects of oxidative stress. In humans, oxidative stress is thought to be involved in the development of many diseases or may exacerbate their symptoms.

The DEFINE trial was the first of two Phase 3 clinical trials to determine the efficacy and safety of BG-12 in people with RRMS. BG-12 BID met the primary and all designated expectations of the trial. It demonstrated a significant reduction in the number of patients who relapsed or had flare-ups. The annual relapse rate was reduced significantly with BG-12 and the risk of disability progression as measured by the Expanded Disability Status Scale at two years compared to patients on the placebo. BG-12 reduced the risk of relapse by 49% reduced the risk of disability progression by 38 %. Magnetic resonance imaging indicated that after two years patients receiving BG-12 experienced significant reductions in the number of brain lesions compared to patients on the placebo.

The CONFIRM trial was the second phase 3 clinical trial and it echoed the findings of the DEFINE trial. Nearly 2600 patients were enrolled in these two trials. The trials spanned over two years.

The most common side effects associated with Tecfidera were flushing, diarrhoea, nausea and abdominal pain. Average lymphocyte counts decreased in some patients during the first year of treatment and then remained stable. Reports of infections and serious infections were similar in Tecfidera-treated patients and those on placebo. Multiple Sclerosis patients taking Tecfidera should have a complete blood count before starting treatment and follow-up tests annually.

BG-12 received Fast Track designation in MS from the U.S. Food and Drug Administration. BG-12 is marketed by Biogen Idec who retains full worldwide commercial rights. It was approved by the FDA, and this will be another Oral Disease Modifying Drug for the treatment of Multiple Sclerosis.

BG-12 is marketed by Biogen Idec under the name Tecfidera.

**Mitoxantrone or Novantrone** has been used to treat Leukemia and prostate cancer. It has been introduced as a treatment for the worst of MS cases, in other words for the following categories of PRMS and SPMS. It is an immune suppressant and clinical trials so far have shown that it is moderately effective in slowing down the relapses in Multiple Sclerosis. It is not approved as a treatment of Relapse Remitting Multiple Sclerosis. The idea behind Novantrone is to suppress the body's immune system and to slow down the immune attacks on the Central Nervous System. Novantrone can be injected every three months for up to three years. Currently that is also the maximum dosage that the FDA has approved.

The presence of other medical problems may affect the use of Novantrone. Let your doctor know if you have any of the following:

- Chicken pox or recent exposure to it

- Herpes zoster (shingles)

- Gout or history of gout

- Kidney stones

- Heart disease

- Liver disease

Common side effects are Nausea, hair loss and menstrual cycle disruptions. Great care most also be taken to reduce the risk of exposure to other diseases, primarily as the body's immune system is being compromised on this treatment. More serious side effects includes fever or chills, lower back or side pain, painful or difficult urination, swelling of feet and lower legs, black, tarry stools, cough or shortness of breath, sores in the mouth or on the lips and stomach pain. Inform your Doctor immediately if you develop these side effects.

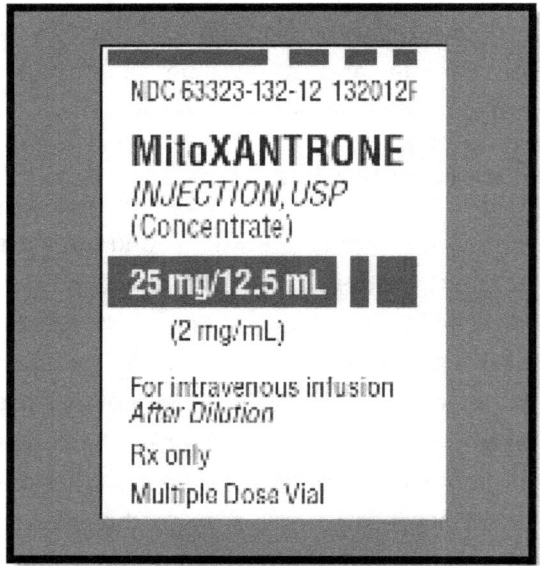

[73] Mitoxantrone (Image source National Library of Medicine (NLM))

Cases of Secondary Acute Myelogenous Leukemia (AML), a type of cancer, have been reported in MS patients and cancer patients treated with Novantrone. Of more serious concern is the risk of heart damage, especially on higher dosages. The cardio toxicity levels of this drug are high and should be given with caution to patients who have underlying heart problems. A proper evaluation needs to be done first before administering the drug.

Novantrone is a chemo therapy drug and will only be prescribed if all other so called "CRAB" drugs fail to slow down the progression in MS.

# Alternative treatments in Multiple Sclerosis.

The new theory is that we have obstructions in our Jugular and Azygos veins, causing a slow perfusion of blood to our brain. I have dealt with this theory earlier on in Dr Zamboni hypothesis and I therefor call this an alternative treatment and not a proven treatment.

Now if we look at the treatment for this condition, the early indication of treatment consists of an angioplasty (placing a balloon in the affected vein to open up these blockages). Another approach was to stent the affected vein (placing a scaffold like device in the vein to keep it open). The first procedure, angioplasty, did not have major complications however 50% of the patient re-stenosed, resulting in them having the procedure redone. The second procedure Stenting; the affected vein seem to last longer, but it had adverse effects like Vagus nerve damages and in one case, stent migration to the heart (This patient needed open heart surgery). Another indirect complication is a fatal stroke caused by the blood thinners. It is however claimed, that it was not directly associated with the procedure but as an unlikely event caused by the blood thinners. However, if the Stenting was not done, the blood thinners probably would not have been needed. (This is just an outside opinion.) This new treatment became known as Liberation treatment.

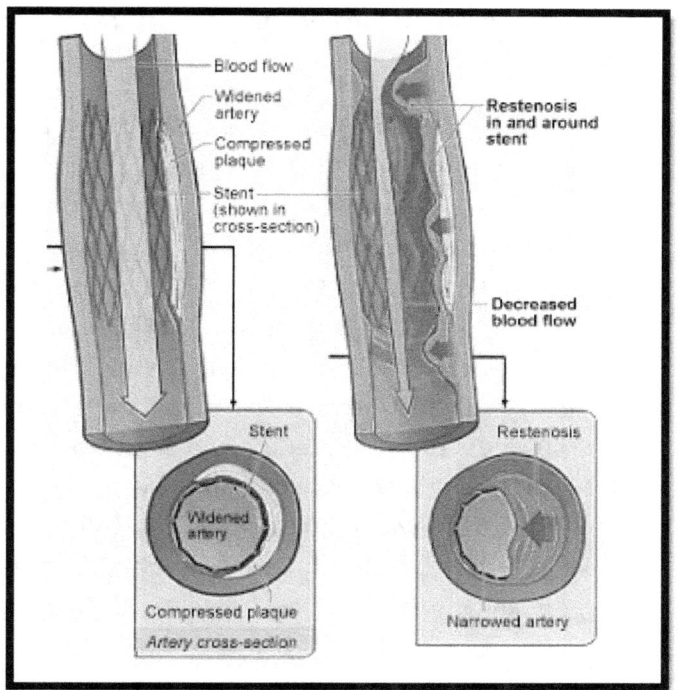

[74] Angioplasty with stenting (Source: National Heart, Lung, and Blood Institute; N I H; U.S. Department of Health and Human Services.)

The initial result of this "Liberation" procedure from what is published, is an immediate effect of decreased fatigue and "brain fog". Another immediate effect is the feeling of warmth in the hands and in the feet, and in some cases, facial colouring. There are also reports of cognitive improvement. There are reports of improvements in balance and bladder problems. Some patients reported improvement in energy levels and increase in muscle strength. The improvement in the EDSS score of patients, is however not remarkable, with an increase of about 1-1.5 points in this regards. There are tracking programs on this over the internet with some patients reporting no benefit from this procedure. This is not totally unexpected, as DR Zamboni published, as it does indicate very little improvements in SPMS and to a lesser extend in PPMS. The biggest benefit was from the RRMS group. But there are also reports of progressing back to pre-liberation condition after a couple of months. It is still too early to tell if this stops the progression of MS or slows it down. Dr Zamboni publishing indicates that it may slow the progression in RRMS, with a 27% relapse as compared to the 50% before liberation.

Lacking though, is the individual study reports on the liberation treatment, and its outcome.

The recent webinar that was conducted by the Multiple Sclerosis society, with the major role players, has reached a consensus that CCSVI and the treatment should be investigated with a certain rigor. There are currently two major studies in the pipeline that will test this theory. Also note that there are a couple of small studies being done as well. The major studies will be done by Buffalo Medical School and the PLLC Vascular group. Both study are very large groups and also have the blessing of NMSS and the respective Ethics committees. The first arm of these studies will test the safety of the "liberation" treatments. This will be a short study. The second arm will study the effectiveness of the procedure and what benefit it creates in Multiple Sclerosis. It will also try to answer some big questions pertaining to this theory. There are many unanswered questions which I will not go into now. In a nutshell, this could be a very big step to a different approach to Multiple Sclerosis and to CCSVI "cause and effect". This could potentially mean big news to Multiple Sclerosis patients.

Unfortunately, it also has some negative responses to this, with patients' shouting "we want this now". This is highly unlikely to happen as it is a new theory and needs rigor in testing. The webinar calls for exactly that, calm until this procedure is tested. I, from my heart, scream "yes I want it now", but reason and sanity tells me that I might not benefit from this, being PPMS and possibly SPMS. The safety protocol of this is not fully proven, as well as the long term benefits or adverse effects. There are reasons that this might have an adverse effect, and the Ethics committees are aware of these. Hence the call for calm, but this will not deter some patients as they feel it is their last option. Now believe me if I say I understand that and so does the researcher. But the role players in this call for exactly that, as this is still very early days.

Then follows the other outrageous claim that it is a vascular disease and thus let the vascular surgeons handles it. This is not the case, as proven; it is a neurological disease with vascular implication. This is similar to strokes, a vascular condition with a neurological implication. Strokes are handled by neurologists and vascular doctors and the same is still true of Multiple Sclerosis. There are still some CCSVI advocates (Note some have objective opinions on it and not all are included) that will make you believe it is purely a vascular condition. Please heed the warning from all the role players, it involves both and to the biggest extend, neurology. And will be so for the next couple of decades until a proven cure is found. However the CCSVI advocates claim that you should hide your diagnosis of MS and go see a doctor claiming headaches and facial pain. The advantage according to them is this: health insurance pays for it and you get the liberation treatment. One, this is very dangerous and can lead to death as certain MS meds do not go well with blood thinners. This is a fact that you will have to keep hidden, putting your health at a major risk.  Two, I wonder if they think that doctors do not read their reference books. They have already caught onto this, and they will not risk their practices by doing this and claim from health insurance. This borderlines on fraud, and they will treat each case on merit, while others have completely shut the door on this. There is a protocol (The Lancet protocol), which is adhered to by vascular surgeons. Hence it will be almost impossible to pursue this avenue, as more and more doctors are shutting down this treatment until the proven trial outcome.

The advocacy groups contend that the governments should make this treatment available. This would be correct if proper trials had taken place. At this stage, it is still a theory and until proven by research, governments will follow the same sensible route of funding trials on the above. Although stenting has been done since 1970, this was only on the arterial side and not the venous side. According to the Lancet protocol, this is done in 50% stenosis with a severe impact on quality of life. If this was said to be true and the avenue governments must follow to improve quality of life, then they should do lung transplant on all emphysema patients. The sad fact is if your Medicaid or Health Insurance does not cover it, they will not add it until it is proven and rubberstamped. At this stage, the quality of life improvement is not yet fully proven, as it could be that 3 years down the line you may end up in a worse condition. Governments and insurances lead themselves by doctors that are the leaders in treating certain conditions, and not individual patient reports. This also applies to vascular diseases. The stumbling block of this is the Lancet protocol, which they will not turn down. Just look back at history; it took about 10 years before angioplasty became a reality. This is a new controversial theory of angioplasty, and needs time to be proven.

Ok say some, "let us as patients take them to court on this and hold protest marches". In the end all they will achieve is questionable. The major (98%) of all vascular and neurological specialists are still very reluctant to do this, until it is proven in trials. In effect, no protest marches will change governments' decisions already taken. They will still go with promoting trials for this. They will call for calm and explain their position on this. In effect, this is already happening. So let us go to litigation? In a lawsuit of this magnitude they will, when it eventually gets to court, which is likely to be 3 years from now, rather side with the majority of professionals, thus shutting down that avenue. A recent lawsuit regarding Autism clearly indicates that fact. Others say, "We have patients to prove this".

Believe me for every one patient that you subpoena to testify, that liberation works, they will put 10 down stating MS medications work. For every doctor that is pro CCSVI, you will have 10 attesting differently. It is a sad state of affairs but this is the reality. Litigation will set CCSVI back at least 5 years, as the indirect cause of this is that even the smaller trials on this might be shut down, by Ethics committees. A similar effect will happen in a congressional hearing as well.

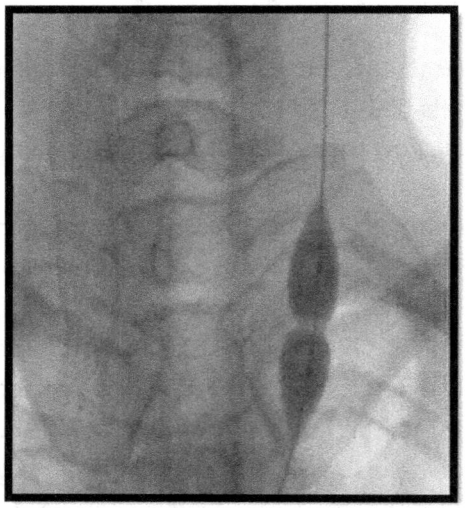

[75] Liberation Treatment (Image source: Wikipedia. Author: Sergei Gutnikov)

The latest scenario, which is happening as we speak, is that with the media hype and the desperation (which is understandable) an ugly result has risen to the surface. In the beginning of CCSVI testing and liberation the cost was about $10k. But like I said, doctors see the response and the advocating on CCSVI sites and the flooding of calls to their surgeries. The adverse effect of this is that they have seen the benefit to them (and that being monetary) hence the reason why the overseas procedure has nearly increased three fold in price. The lowest price for liberation internationally is $10k and rising up to $100k and more. This will happen, and the price is likely to continue to rise. However I cannot include all doctors that perform this procedure; in this mix there is one or two that have the patient in mind and not their wallet. There are also doctors that claim that they are trained by the pioneer of this procedure. Some of these are false claims as stated by Dr Zamboni. A further scenario is that scammers are latching onto this as well. So be very cautious of this.

Should we allow compassionate access to Liberation treatment? "Yes" as Dr Zamboni states, but it should be done on a patient review basis and not on a word of mouth from the patient. In other words, if you have exhausted all of the other avenues this must be made available as a last resort. But the last resort must be just that, you have tried all the meds and stayed on course with your treatments and it is progressing badly. Do not use the fact of not complying with using DMD as an excuse to seek this route. This is totally unethical, as it will take resources away from some patients that have no other options, while you have the choice to take DMD but you refused use them. Then you will have those that say "I am not putting that poison in my system", but I want this treatment as compassion. That is not compassionate access, but rather selfish access.

In my opinion CCSVI is a big issue that needs rigor in research, but we, as the patients must help to make this happen. Help with funding, for those that can afford it, but don't take away from current research. Make others aware of this without imposing ridiculous claims on this with a statement that it is a cure and the only route to go. This is not needed, as about 50% will not benefit from this. It is still not a cure, but at best, a new treatment for a symptom of MS. It will probably benefit about 50% of patients, while certainly not all. Could it be the cause of MS, highly unlikely, but it could definitely be a complication of MS. It could also be an explanation why some progress faster than others. Could it stop progression, perhaps yes or could it slow it down? That question will remain unanswered for at least 10 years.

CCSVI is new hope for MS Patients but it is still in its infancy. I have hopes that through sensible actions, this can become a reality as a new treatment and open new avenues of research on Multiple Sclerosis. But I am not putting all my eggs in that basket yet.

## Possible complications in Liberation treatment.

A question recently asked; "What is the possible complication if you re-stenosed"? Now I trust this is an open source document as it is posted on several sites, and if it is not, then I do apologize in advance. The answer was supplied by Dr Simka from Poland. I am just highlighting the points raised and will quote the relevant sections.

Dr Simka states that the possibility of restenosis is real and in certain cases it has happened. This is also evident from the reports from patients who have re-stenosed. In the case of balloon angioplasty, this is not such a big complication as the vein can be reopened. The number of times is still uncertain, but from all whom I had discussions with, chances are that eventually vein damage will happen. But in the case of Stenting, a new problem does arise. In most case this can be reopened but, and in certain cases if the stent is completely blocked, it is unlikely to reopen it, and the stent will have to be removed. Unfortunately there is only one way of removing the stent and that is to surgically remove it out of the vein. In the case of jugular, it will mean opening the neck which may not have many complications but in case of the Azygos, it involves major surgery.

I quote the section from Dr Simka's letter.

"Regarding the treatment, we opt for the safest and the most efficient treatment, which of course is not possible, since those two parameters don't meet it every case. Balloon angioplasty has already been demonstrated to be very safe in a short time, and most likely safety in long time is also nearly perfect. But balloon angioplasty is not very efficacious. In some cases it doesn't work at all, in the others there are late restenoses. The short-term efficacy of an alternative treatment - stenting is much higher. But long-term efficacy (risk of late occlusion) is not known. Although an occluded stent can be opened, but probably not in every case. And of course there are known early complications related to stents, namely the migrations that exclude some anatomic variants from stenting (at least using currently available stents). There is also possible the open repair of the vein, but risk and efficacy of such procedures are not known. Thus, all treatment modalities should be regarded as experimental, with still unknown efficacy and safety. The doctors always try to balance the risk and the efficacy factors, but the best solution is not always possible and is not always chosen (importantly, we don't have data on long term consequences of ballooning or stenting)."

Dr Simka's answer on whether "Liberation Treatment" is a cure for MS is also a very clear.  He is clearly of the opinion that MS is not CCSVI, but that MS could be CCSVI and some other factors. My opinion because CCSVI (Buffalo study) is not found in all patients, CCSVI is rather a complication of MS, or a contributing factor to MS progression.

I quote that section from Dr Simka letter.

"CCSVI is not an equivalent for MS; most likely, MS = CCSVI + some (probably more than one) other factors"

"Consequently, treating CCSVI does not mean that MS is gone. Most of the patients experience good and bad days following surgery, importantly, during infection, stress, etc. the symptoms usually go back. But the symptoms also go back in a case of restenosis."

Does "Liberation Treatment" benefit all MS patients? According to Dr Simka this is not the case in all, with some not receiving any benefits, while others had worsening of their MS. There are also cases where this has happened even with successful stenting or balloon angioplasty. But it has the best benefits still in RRMS patients. But the chance of restenosis is still there and it does happen.

Again I quote that section from Dr Simka's letter.

"Treatment of CCSVI does not guarantee improvement. There were some patients (not much, still, they were) who experienced worsening. Most of those patients presented with severely narrowed veins that could not be sufficiently managed with ballooning or stenting, but there were also cases with "perfectly" done surgery. So, a patient can improve after surgery (a majority, especially relapsing remitting patients), but no improvement or even worsening is also possible. A reoperation can improve the symptoms in the latter two groups, but again, not in all cases."

"Probably, surgery for CCSVI + pharmaceutical treatment will improve outcomes. Try to continue your neurological medication if it were working before surgery. "

Thus my summary of the above, the long term benefits as well as complications are still not known and there is still a great and urgent need for controlled studies on this. Personally I do understand why patient feel that this may be a last option or hope, and travel these distances to have the procedure done, but I just need to add this caution and also a reason why you should rather opt for go-local if you can. And also heed the warning of this stay on your MS meds as going off them may have dire consequences to your health in certain cases.

A fact that needs to be mentioned, and cannot be ignored, is the ethics behind CCSVI and "Liberation Treatment". In essence Doctor Zamboni's ethical position has been questioned. Of note is the fact that his own wife is afflicted by Multiple Sclerosis and some are calling his objectivity into question.

**My own personal feeling about CCSVI.**

Well, it has been nearly three years since the media storms erupted around the discovery of Dr Paulo Zamboni and Chronic Cerebro Spinal Venous Insufficiency, and there are very mixed reports and results thus far over the new possible treatment called "Liberation". There are strong advocates for CCSVI and also strong anti CCSVI advocates. Some new trials have also been implemented to test this theory and more trials are also called for. Patient are lobbying strongly for the treatment as well as some influential persons in governments also calling for further research in this area, as well as some doctors.  Patients are reporting in blogs, web and social pages about their experiences as well and their results after "Liberation". Now please don't shoot the messenger, but the messenger is reading what is out there and his interpretation of it, is an unbiased opinion.

The messenger's opinion is that there is a place for CCSVI in Multiple Sclerosis and it may certainly benefit us, but to what extend we do not know, but my hopes are high that eventually it will increase the quality of life for some of us. Whether it is a cure I think only time will tell, but I would not label it as such, but rather a complication and a new possible treatment for Multiple Sclerosis, especially in the beginning stage. "Are we looking at a new cause of the disease, being vascular and not an Auto-immune disease?" I think it is too soon to jump to that conclusion as Multiple Sclerosis has all the classical markers of an Auto-immune disease and in fact, research has proven this for the better part of the last fifty plus years. But it could be a new complication that can affect the disease course in many patients. Vascular connection has been studied over the last 50 plus years as well, but never before was such an interesting discovery made.

CCSVI has an important role to play in Multiple Sclerosis, and the various patients that report an improvement in the symptoms of the disease is a very good sign for this important new development. Most of the Relapse Remitting Multiple Sclerosis patients do report a good measure of improvement, and this lent weight to this new theory. In the case of progressive Multiple Sclerosis (SPMS and PPMS) the improvements are not that great, with most reporting little or no benefit, but this is to a certain extent expected as the damage that Multiple Sclerosis can cause is extensive, with nerve endings in the brain and spinal cord being permanently damaged or lost. We might be at the dawn of a new era in the treatment of Multiple Sclerosis, especially for the newly diagnosed patient, in the beginning stages of Multiple Sclerosis and this new treatment might just hold a new promise to them of slowing down the progression of the disease, and could even benefit some of us old timers as well.

Lacking though, are any long term results that can shed more light on the subject, but this is not surprising as any new treatment in medical time can take from 2- 20 years to prove or disprove itself. Patients are outraged, wanting this treatment now and refuse to wait, but this is expected as Multiple Sclerosis is a disease that drives fear into a person living with it. This has given the rise to MS organizations calling for calm until this theory is proven or debunked as such, but as with any fear driven disease, patients flew all over the world to have this treatment done. This is also expected and in my opinion, certain patients feel that this is their last hope and we cannot fault them for this, as they are facing a future with the probability of being disabled or are already disabled from Multiple Sclerosis. Preliminary reports indicate that it will benefit certainly the Relapsing Remitting Multiple Sclerosis patients and to a lesser extend the Progressive Multiple Sclerosis group (PPMS or SPMS). Labelling this as a placebo affect seems a bit far fetch and his figures do warrant more extensive trials.

Now the big question:" Will the theory hold or will it die a thousand deaths at the end of all the research?" My own opinion so far is that it will certainly benefit some patients but there may also be certain complications in this treatment. Searching through all the patient pages, there is a strong indication that we might have a new form of treatment for Multiple Sclerosis, but it looks at this stage that it is only a treatment that may improve the quality of life of certain patients, and may slow down the disease to a certain extent. Dr Zamboni's initial figures indicate that about 50% will have their jugular and Azygos veins narrowing up again in the first year to 18 months. Considering that most of his results are published on RRMS patients, it is difficult to tell if this is the due to the natural course of Multiple Sclerosis. Most RRMS patients tend to relapse very little during the initial 5-10 years after the onset of Multiple Sclerosis and can go into remission for a long period of time. But added to that, his figures do point to a relative success rate in about 27% of his group. But what constitutes this percentage? Are these patients that can go without relapse for 3 years or more? These are questions that can only be answered by long term studies and more published results.

Reading all the patient pages, it seems that most report an improvement of "brain fog", eyesight and energy and some reporting balance and gait improvement. The improvement on the Expanded Disability Status Scale being reported is at around 1 point, but again these are patient reports and not actual medical reports. The most outstanding report is the feeling of warm hands and feet immediately after "Liberation". Some patients report very little or no improvement, with some reporting only improvement after a couple of weeks. Most patients do not report relapses, but some do and in certain cases it is attributed to collapsing of the veins. Certain cases of relapses cannot be tied to collapsing or narrowing of the veins again, with patients reporting that no restenosis of the vein were found and it seems at this stage, that you can relapse without restenosis of the veins. Sadly, there are also reports of being worse off after the procedure and this a bit of a concern. This is not openly reported by the CCSVI advocates, but the reports are on the web and it is a matter of finding them. They are few but they are still out there.

There are however, the other side of reports which sound a little far-fetched, but these are a very few patient reports and it is not known if we must take this with a "pinch of salt" or are there actual improvements. I am not inclined to point blank shoot these down but, certain reports of patients climbing out of their wheelchairs and walking afterwards, does tend to let me to err somewhat on the side of caution. With Multiple Sclerosis widespread muscle atrophy is one of the leading causes why patients end up in a wheelchair, and a "liberation" will not result in you getting up and walking immediately afterwards. These patients will need weeks of physical therapy to regain the muscle strength to walk again. This is all too apparent in brain injury and spinal cord patients who are temporarily disabled and also need physical therapy to build strength in the legs and to be able to walk again. The only conclusion that can be drawn from this assumption, and I apologise for being very straight forward here, is perhaps sensationalising and attention seeking from these patients. Whatever the case is, liberation will not result in a miracle "I can walk again", as this goes against any medical evidence. This can only be believed if, in a case where the patient underwent physical therapy afterwards, but that gives rise to a new question. "Is it a case of practice builds strength or is the actual strength regained from Liberation?" This is another question that needs to be answered by further studies.

Getting back to the feeling of warm hands and feet, this was noted by Dr Simka a pioneer in the field of CCSVI as perhaps an Angiotensin effect. Angiotensin is a peptide hormone that causes vasoconstriction and a subsequent increase in blood pressure. Angiotensin II is responsible for the body's temperature, and altering the blood flow to the brain can increase this, hence explaining the feeling of warm hands and feet. As for the general feeling of wellbeing it could be a direct result of "Liberation" and repairing the blood from the brain, stopping the reflux of oxygen poor blood in the brain. But again, we need a lot of studies in this area, as Angiotensin could also play a role in this as well. This is not only my feeling, but is also the feeling of Dr Simka. Fatigue in Multiple Sclerosis has still a relatively unknown cause, and correcting the blood flow from the ventricles in the brain could certainly have an effect on this, but the fact that some patient report an immediate improvement of "brain fog" and energy directly after the liberation procedure could rather be attributed to Angiotensin effect as well. Correcting the blood flow does not result in the immediate removal of all excess iron and immediate repair of the damage done by Multiple Sclerosis, but would rather take a couple weeks to change. Altering the blood flow volume can alter or increase the function of the hypothalamus or the part of the brain that is responsible for most neuro-hormone production. This in turn, could lead to the increase of ACTH, ADH, neuro-pinephrines and dopamine levels, leading to the feeling of wellbeing. However, a large percentage of patients who did have the procedure eventually lose this feeling after a couple of months without re-stenosing. Certain patients actually report this feeling of new lease of life and increase energy only after a couple of weeks, and this could be interpreted as a direct result of "Liberation treatment". A direct result of the treatment as well is the fact that balance, gait and strength improves after a couple of weeks in some patients.

Lastly the question: "Is this procedure safe, and are there long term complications?" Balloon angioplasty is relatively safe, and there is little complication to report. If one leads oneself by the USA national figures for angioplasty, there is a 2-6% severe complication rate, some leading to death, but I must add that this figure is based on all angioplasty, and the bulk of these complications are reported in heart and stroke patients. However, it seems that the complication is rather less in CCSVI as the procedure is more on the venous side and not the arterial side.

The first report is of a stent migrating causing open heart surgery, and the tragic death of Holly. Holly's death was attributed to a stroke and not as a result of the procedure, but the complication was enough to stop Stanford doing the procedures. But new reports have surfaced on Multiple Sclerosis sites of blood clots developing in a couple of patients, and in a few cases, the clots were severe enough to either cause a lung embolism or a stroke. Fortunately it was caught in time and the patients were spared from suffering a severe complication. Most of these clots were reported where the patients had stents implanted. A further complication that has also arisen is the occlusion of the stent and in three cases, open neck surgery was required to remove the stent and the cloth. In other cases, the stent was successfully opened by means of re-angioplasty. But this is serious enough to warrant further investigation in the use of stents etc. A further complication is the rate of restenosis where stents are not used, and continual ballooning may eventually lead to further complications.

With all the above being said, there is a definite need to further investigate CCSVI and the procedure to correct this. As Dr Simka stated, CCSVI is not the direct cause of Multiple Sclerosis, but rather CCSVI and other factors. In my mind, the only ultimate theory is that Multiple Sclerosis is an Auto-immune disease and CCSVI is rather a complication from the disease and not the cause of it. Treating CCSVI may certainly benefit the bulk of RRMS patients, or compliment the current treatment as we know it. In my opinion, we will have to wait for the next round of trials that are currently in the pipeline, before we jump to unnecessary conclusions on this important discovery. Let us all hope that this leads to at least a better understanding of Multiple Sclerosis, or as duped by some the "Mystery Sickness", and keep the messenger intact as he might still have something important to say.

**Low Dose Naltrexone** (LDN) has been suggested and is advocated as a treatment for Multiple Sclerosis. The Multiple Sclerosis Centre at UCSF has recently completed a double blind, placebo crossover trial on the benefits of Low Dose Naltrexone (LDN) on Multiple Sclerosis patients to evaluate the effectiveness of this drug. 80 patients enrolled in the trial but only 60 completed the trial. The objective was to test the effectiveness of LDN as proclaimed by MS patients. The trial was over an 8 week period to see the impact on Quality of Life in Ms Patients on LDN. The dropout rate of 25% had a significant impact on results of the trail, and impeded a bit on the statistical data. Bruce Cree, MD and co-researchers at the Multiple Sclerosis Centre at University of California, San Francisco, published their study "Pilot Trial Of Low Dose Naltrexone and Quality of Life in MS" in the online journal of the Annals of Neurology on February 19, 2010.

Naltrexone is an opioid receptor antagonist or in plain English; it blocks effects of opioids on the brain. It is marketed in generic form as its hydrochloride salt, naltrexone hydrochloride, and marketed under the trade names Revia and Depad. Low-dose naltrexone (LDN) is an "off-label" use of the medication naltrexone at low doses for Multiple Sclerosis. Naltrexone is typically prescribed for opioid dependence or alcohol dependence. The trial being a cross over trial, meaning that the patient was switched after a wash out period from placebo to LDN and vice versa. This was also a paid patient trial. There were very few adverse events and minor events were as follows.

1. Vivid dreams (8 placebos and 10 LDN)

2. Fatigue (2 placebos and 1 LDN)

3. Flu-like symptoms (1 placebo)

4. Insomnia (1 placebo)

5. Loss of appetite (1 LDN)

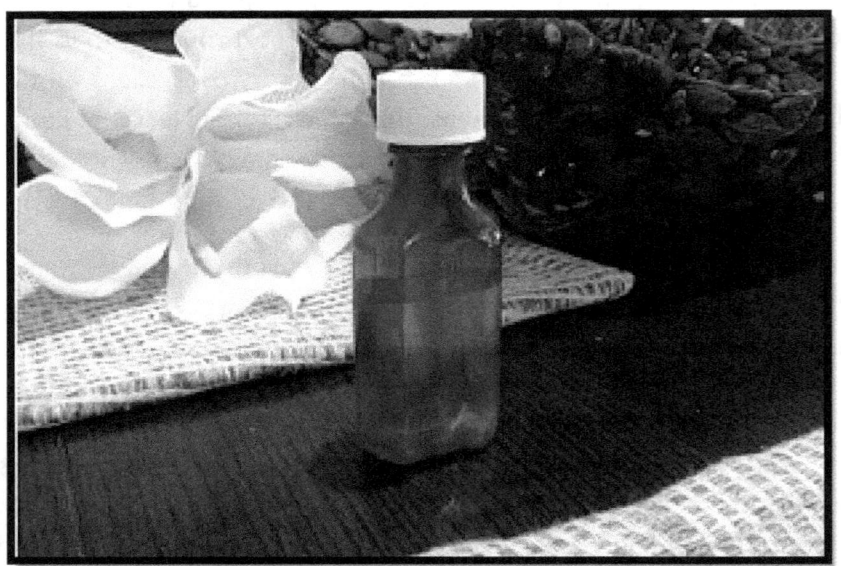

[76] Naltrexone (Image Courtesy of Brittany Garcia)

No relapse was reported during the period of the trial, but this is not a good measure to test the effect on relapse, as the trial was over a short span. The mental health outcome was reported to have improved over the short span of this trial, indicating that LDN has the ability to improve the patient's mental skills. This is also conclusive with the anecdotal reports of patient feeling better after using LDN. The researcher concluded that LDN may have an effect on the Endorphin levels of patients thus explaining the feeling of mental well-being. However in this trial, LDN has not shown an increase in the physical impact of the patient. As there were only 8 weeks of treatment in this trial this is to be expected. The same correlation can also be drawn in DMD's as the immediate benefits are highly unlikely to be proven in 8 weeks.

On the physical outcome of Quality of life, there was no significant difference between the start of the trial and the completion. The EDSS of patients were not measured in this trial as the trial was relatively short.

The effect of LDN on the mental health component score compares favourably to that of Tysabri suggesting that the magnitude of difference relative to placebo for this measure is clinically relevant (a 3.3 point increase at 8 weeks for LDN compared to a 1.0 to 2.5 point increase at 2 years for Tysabri). This benefit for LDN treatment was supported by significant improvements on the mental health scale. On the pain effects scale there was an increase of about 0.8 points. In DMD's this scale has not been measured as such and therefore this value at this stage is purely statistical.

However since LDN is not suggested to replace DMD's, the benefit of LDN is only intended to be a symptomatic treatment on the "Quality of Life" in Multiple Sclerosis.

What can be concluded from this trial is that LDN has shown an impact on the Mental Quality of life, but the trial was too short to measure the Physical quality of life, but evidence does exist to further studies on LDN in Multiple Sclerosis.

**Stem Cell treatment In Multiple Sclerosis.**

The University of Bristol in the United Kingdom has completed a Phase I Trial on Stem cell treatment in Multiple Sclerosis and published their findings. The study results were published one year after the trail started to measure the effect on Multiple Sclerosis. Six patients having Multiple Sclerosis ranging from 9 to 20 years participated in this trial. The Expanded Disability Scale of this patient range from 4.5 to 6.5 in this trail.

Rather than targeting specific bone marrow cells the researcher decided to opt for whole bone marrow transplant. In the past certain target specific stem cell procedures did not show, therefore the decision, for whole bone marrow cell transplants. The patient's bone marrow was removed and filtered. After this process it was added to the patient by means of an IV infusion. The procedure did not require an overnight stay in hospital, and one patient suffered urine retention and two had an increase in lower limb spasticity post infusion. Over all the treatment was received well and none had a serious adverse event.

In the twelve month follow up period, one patient had a relapse two months after the procedure, but the rest remained stable for the period. On the EDSS scale, only one patient had a decrease of 0.5 points while the rest remained the same. No significant improvement was reported over the one year period. However, the researchers were encouraged by the increase of the global evoked potentials, which started showing improvement after 3 months and were sustained for the rest of the year. However, they point out that since there were a small number of patients and no controls; firm conclusions cannot be drawn about the effectiveness of the procedure.

But what is encouraging with this treatment is that it could perhaps halt MS progression and more specific treatments in future could even lead to a decrease in MS Symptoms. Ultimately, this type of stem cell treatment indicated that it may be a safe procedure and a larger control trial is now planned. But this has ratified what the MS societies have said in their guidelines that stem cell treatment is still not a cure, but a hope for future treatment of Multiple Sclerosis.

According to a new study conducted in 2012 by the University of Rochester Medical Centre (URMC) the ability to manipulate the brain into manufacturing an endless supply of oligodendrocytes, which produce myelin is possible. The focus of this study is on the glial progenitor cells (GPCs) that are found in the white matter of the brain. According to the researchers : "These stem cells give rise to two cells found in the central nervous system: oligodendrocytes, which produce myelin, the fatty tissue that insulates the connections between cells; and astrocytes, cells that are critical to the health and signalling function of oligodendrocytes as well as neurons." Having the ability to reproduce myelin in the brain, can certainly benefit all the diseases were Myelin damage is the root cause of the disease.

The only problem with this experiment was the ability to stop Myelin growth once it has been started. Again I quote: "However, after a period of time this process slows and, instead of replicating, the cells begin to then commit to becoming one type or another. The challenge for scientists was to find another way to essentially trick these cells into continuing to divide, and to do so without risking the uncontrolled growth that could otherwise result in tumor formation."

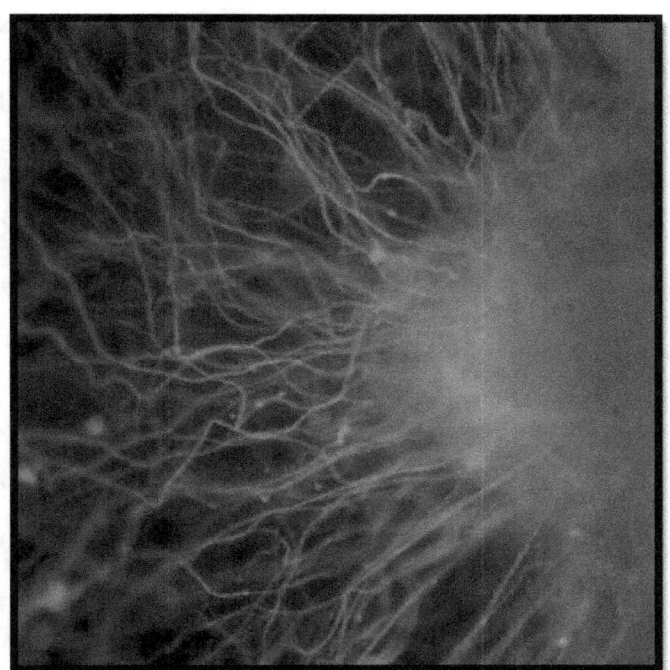

[77] Stem Cell Reproduction (Image source: Wikipedia. Author: Nissim Benvenisty)

The study used brain stem cells for the experiment, but recognises the ability to grow this stem cell from human skin or embryotic cells.

I quote from the NMSS official website.

"Researchers have agreed that stem cells are likely to have a significant role to play in the treatment of MS, but also warn that expectations should be realistic." Professor Gianvito Martino said, "At this stage it is unreasonable to claim that stem cells are a magic cure for MS. It is, however, likely that they will one day play an important role in treating the condition."

Although stem cell treatment is not officially recognised as a treatment for Multiple Sclerosis, it is highly advocated and is offered as a treatment in certain countries. The current belief by some patients and advocacy groups are that stem cell treatment can cure MS to an extent or halt the disease. There are also lobbyists for the simultaneous use of stem cell treatment coupled with "Liberation Treatment", and believes this will be the treatment of most, if not all, of our MS symptoms, with some even calling it the new cure.

**The Swank Diet** was introduced in 1948 by Doctor Roy L Swank (1909-2008). His book, The Multiple Sclerosis Diet Book, has achieved wide attraction from both within and outside the medical community. However his study was widely criticised over the years, questioning his methods and other similar research that was done on Polyunsaturated Fatty Acids (PUFA's) over the years could not prove the diet actually works.

Dr Swank diet consists basically of

- Saturated fat should not exceed 15 grams per day

- Unsaturated fat should be kept to 20-50 grams per day

- No red meat for the first year; after that, a maximum of 3 oz. (85 grams) of red meat per week

- Dairy products must contain 1% or less butterfat

- No processed foods containing saturated fat

- A good source of omega-3 (oily fish, cod liver oil, cod liver oil tablets, etc.) along with a multi-vitamin and mineral supplement are recommended daily

- Wheat, gluten or dairy product quantities are not restricted. But foods which cause allergies or reactions to an MS sufferer should be avoided

The above is the basis for his diet. I just need to elaborate on the last one a bit. Back in the 1940's some Doctors still believed that MS was caused by an allergic reaction, therefor the last caution.

DR swank was also one of the firm believers that MS is caused by a vascular disease.

His initial study was based on Norwegian findings that MS is more common in the mountainous regions than the coastal areas. Based on this, he concluded that those living in the mountain were more exposed to satirised fat like butter, cheese and milk as compared to the coast with more fish and seafood. Professor Monrad

Krohn, Chief of Neurology, noted that he seldom saw cases of MS from along the coast, where fishing was the primary industry, but further inland, and in the mountains, the frequency of MS was more common.

Now this is a point we need to dwell on a bit. Looking at Norway and taking into account the behaviour of people, we could ultimately come to a different conclusion today. The prevalence of MS at the coast in Oslo was 1 in 10 000, whereas inland it was 9 in 10 000 although these figures have never been verified. Now anybody that lives at the coast will note that people are more prone to sun exposure than inland, and in the 1940s, Norway's primary industry was fishing, hence even more sun exposure. One needs to only look at the fishermen and note the sun and sea damage on their skin. Also there is a tendency of persons visiting the beach more often than those inland. Oslo in itself is also further south than inland, and the UV index is higher. Taking the above into account, it does not rate diet as the sole influence on MS numbers in Norway, but rather geographical and climate conditions need to be taken into account as well. Note NARCOMS and the correlations of other databases for MS patients put the figure in Norway at 4.2 – 4.5 patients per 10 000, which is far less than the study from Dr Krohn.

Another factor include in his writings is that German speaking patients had higher incidences of Multiple Sclerosis than Italian speaking patients in Switzerland. Now I am never going to go into language as a cause of MS, as this would be totally absurd.  The presumption here is that Germans eat more fatty food than Italians. Again we go to geographical influences. The tally among Germans is 3.9 – 4-2 per 10 000 compared to 3.0 – 3-6 depending on how far south in Italy. Based on the fact that the theory exists and is proven to an extend that MS develops in the first 15 years of your life, it cannot be concluded with absolute certainty that it is a direct result of being deprived of fatty foods in the Second World War. It would rather suggest that again, geographical and hereditary influences play a role in this assumption.

We only need to look at Northern Colorado and the Rocky Mountain region to understand how an important geographical influence has on MS numbers. The incidences here are high compared to the rest of the USA with an estimated 8.4 out of 10 000 diagnosed with it. We can draw a direct conclusion to this geographical location. Exposure to sunlight in this area is limited due to snow and high altitude. The normal prevalence is 3.6 to 4.2 for every 10 000.

In 1950 Dr swank started his study with 144 patients over a period of 34 years in Montreal. The study in itself is called into question. There were no double blinding studies done, as in the case with a proper study. No proper evaluations were ever carried out and the main source of information was supplied by the patients themselves. The publications are also very vague and yes, 70% did live after 40 years of the study, but the mean onset ages were never published. The remaining patients who passed away, is said to be of none MS related causes, however there is no medical evidence to prove or disprove this. What must also be noted from DR Swank suggestions and these include:

- Sufficient rest with a nap in the afternoon.

- Avoid Stress

- Avoid heat.

This in itself will also benefit Multiple Sclerosis.

The later studies found that even though the diet may play a part in Multiple Sclerosis, the benefits are very little. Fish oil like Omega 3 can have an impact on your Multiple Sclerosis. However there have been countless studies on diet in Multiple Sclerosis, but still no clear link is found.

Now comes the big question; "Can we benefit from a diet". Any disease can and will benefit from a proper balanced diet. Heart healthy diets are good for any person. However, avoid the pitfalls of people offering books and so called diet cures for Multiple Sclerosis. No diet can and will cure Multiple Sclerosis, period, and any neurologist will confirm this. But some say, neurologists are getting kickbacks to supply medications. Now this is the most absurd statement out there. If diet alone was certain to better MS, it would have been long practiced.

**Apitherapy** is the medical use of honey bee products. This includes the use of honey, pollen, bee bread, propolis, royal jelly, apilarnil, and bee venom. It is widely advocated as a cure for Multiple Sclerosis with some websites dedicated to this treatment.

An estimate of about 5000 patients has used this therapy, suggesting that it does help them. Bee sting therapy consist of about 20-40 stings at a time, for three sessions a week. The bees are held by tweezers against the body with the stingers to the skin. The stingers are then held in for about 15 minutes at a time. This is normally done by trained persons. Firstly, the patient needs to be tested for an allergic reaction to bee venom. By injecting the patent with a weak dosage of bee venom, they can determine if you are allergic or not. However you may not be allergic to a small dosage, but could be for a large amount and it may result in anaphylaxis shock, which may ultimately lead to your sudden demise.

The theory behind Bee Sting Therapy is rather simple. By causing an inflammatory reaction to the bee sting area, the inflammatory reaction that causes a Myelin attack is redirected to the bee sting area. This shift in focus reduces the body's immune response to a flare up in a typical relapse. It is also used by patients with many different autoimmune disorders, rheumatoid arthritis, lupus and scleroderma. Bee Sting Therapy is used for a number of other diseases and conditions, including depression, skin conditions, menstrual cramps and varicose veins. There are many risk factors involved in this therapy as well:

- Death: A small number of people (less than 100) die every year from reactions to bee stings.

- Optic Neuritis: This inflammation of the optic nerve has been caused in people, even without MS being reported

- Acute Disseminated Encephalomyelitis: This is a rare form of inflammation of the Central Nervous System.

Bee Sting Therapy should not be used by people with insulin-dependent diabetes or diseases like syphilis, gonorrhoea, tuberculosis or severe allergies. Bee Sting Therapy is also very painful and adding ice to the actual sting area may help.

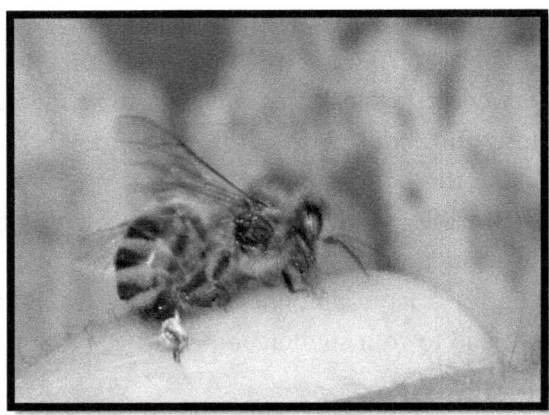

[78] Bee Sting Therapy. (Image source: Wikipedia, Author: Waugsberg)

Now the big question, does it work? In this writer's opinion and almost all neurologists this claim is absolute rubbish. It is also medically been proven that it does not benefit MS at all and in fact it could worsen your Multiple Sclerosis. A couple of trials have been done in animals and a very small phase one trial on humans. There were absolutely no benefits for the disease. However, about 1300 patients have sent in testimonials to the Apitherapy Society, that it does actually decrease fatigue and spasticity, and helps with stability. This represents less than 1.3 in every 10000 patients. And none of these testimonials are supported by any medical based information. And I am willing to bet my last dollar that, if these 1300 patients are queried again in ten years' time, most will sing a completely different tune. In 2004 a randomized crossover study was conducted in Netherlands among 24 patients with either relapsing-remitting MS or secondary-progressive MS. The treatment was well-tolerated but no beneficial effects were seen among these patients.

Would I suggest Bee Sting Therapy for Multiple Sclerosis? My answer "If you want to waste your money and enjoy pain then go for it. Plus you may perhaps risk your life as well." It is a complete bunch of hogwash in my honest opinion. It is advocated by money grabbers who have your wallet in mind and not your health.

**Medical marijuana** is used as an alternative treatment in Multiple Sclerosis. Now for those of you in the dark, this is cannabis or the good old "joint" as it was called in my younger years. This treatment has caused major debates in the last couple of years, with those for the use of it and those against it; "It is an illegal Drug". Yes that it is in most countries, but it is being legalised all over the world for use in certain diseases. Let us not lose focus here; opiates, the major component of schedule six drugs like morphine is made of synthetic cocaine, but in the earlier years of medicine these pain killers consisted of opium, poppy straw concentrate, and other poppy derivatives.

So this is now the catch 22 situation, it does work in Multiple Sclerosis, but it is illegal. But so was opium in the early 1900, but it was prescribed like candy. Luckily governing bodies like the Food and Drug Administration do exist, and in most USA and Canadian states it is now being legalised for medical use. The FDA guidance has been followed for years and has a major input as to what can be used and what not. The rest of the world normally follow suit on their recommendations.

In a small crossover study that was conducted and published in the Canadian Medical Association Journal it was suggested that it does help with pain and spasticity in MS. The study consisted of 30 patients who had either the real deal or a placebo, which looked and tasted like marijuana. The outcome of this study was that it definitely benefited patients with MS. Participants on the real deal showed a 30% improvement in spasticity, compared to those on the placebo. The pain levels in this group drop by a whopping 5.28 points. The only drawback was the increase in fatigue and dizziness and reduced cognitive function. Larger trials are now being called for.

Medical marijuana has been in use for thousands of years as an herbal remedy by traditional healers and medicine men in the past. However that being said, I guess here is to where we call; "To each his own". Sativex is very similar to marijuana and has shown the same benefits, with far less side effects, and a reduction in addictiveness. However a lot of other drugs that we do take can certainly cause similar side effects as marijuana.

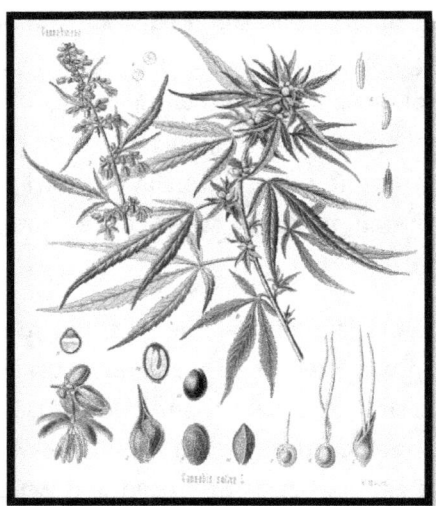

[79] Medical marijuana

I would certainly not shoot this one down as a treatment, although I would rather opt for the safer drugs like Sativex if needed. As with pure Medical marijuana, the same counts for Sativex, there are certain legal barriers to cross.

**Chelation therapy** in Multiple Sclerosis is not a new thing and has been known for decades. Chelation therapy consists of administrating of chelating agents to remove heavy metals from the body. The use of Mercury fillings in dentistry gave rise to the idea that mercury poisoning was directly involved in the onset of MS, blaming Mercury poisoning as a possible cause for MS and other neurological disorders. This resulted in many MS patients removing these fillings. This has never been proven although a tiny amount of Mercury could land in the bloodstream the levels were way too low to have an impact on your health. Again there are strong advocates for this and strong advocates against this, however the use of Mercury has seldom been used in dentistry for a couple of decades and there has been no significant drop in the prevalence of Multiple Sclerosis. There is also no clear study that indicates that Mercury is the cause of Multiple Sclerosis.

Chelation therapy has a long been used for the most common forms of heavy metal intoxication, those involving lead, arsenic or mercury. This is the standard treatment of heavy metal poisoning and a range of chelating agents is available.

However the amount of mercury in dentistry does not need the attention of such aggressive treatments. Chelation therapy is either administered in pill form or intravenously. The mention of Mercury as a potential cause for Multiple Sclerosis, led to clinics popping up overnight to remove the mercury and other heavy medal toxins, like lead from paint, out of our systems. They had a brief existence until the FDA and other medical regulatory bodies stepped in to stop this myth.

It was practiced in moderation for years in countries that do allow it, and this was a hope for some MS patients out there. But by the announcement on CCSVI and the increase of iron deposits found in the brain, this idea hit the headlines again. With diseases that drive fear into many of MS patients, advocacy groups jumped up again proclaiming that the removal of the excess iron deposit in the brain can "cure" Multiple Sclerosis. The suggestion was that "Liberation Treatment" together with Chelation Therapy can ultimately reduce the impact of MS on our lives. This is so far void from the truth as with any brain damage, stroke, brain trauma or disease like Multiple Sclerosis or Parkinson, there is an increase in iron deposits as a direct by-product from axonal death. To put in plain English, dying brain cells leave a trail of iron behind.

The sad reality is again, patients spending thousands of dollars on a treatment that has never been proven to work for Multiple Sclerosis. Again the clinics advocating these treatments, are shouting from the rooftops about this to fill their wallets, and have actually little concern for your health. There are very strong warnings from the FDA and other medical protection agencies that this is a dangerous form of treatment and you could end up on a slab in the morgue long before your time.

Chelation Therapy is only to be used in actual cases of heavy metal poisoning, to save a life as a result from industrial exposure, or the actions of a jealous spouse trying to "off" their partner.

**Green tea extract** is one of these. Green tree extract is an ancient remedy used by the Chinese for centuries and has certainly a number of benefits. Green tea is one of the most practical cancer preventives, as was shown in various studies.

Epigallocatechin gallate (EGCG) is found in green tea but also in rooibos tea and is a potent anti-oxidant that may have therapeutic applications in the treatment of many disorders like cancer. EGCG is a natural chelation agent and has been shown to reduce iron-accumulation in instances of neurodegenerative diseases like dementia, Alzheimer's, and Parkinson's. A recent study has shown that neuro-protective and neuro-regenerative effects could be seen in the animal model, where combination treatment with EGCG and Glatiramer acetate significantly delayed disease onset, reduced clinical severity and reduced inflammatory infiltrates. This study indicates the promise of combining neuro-protective and anti-inflammatory treatments and strengthens the prospects of Green Tee Extract as an added therapy for neuro-inflammatory and neuro-degenerative diseases. However, this has never been tested in MS alone, but together with Glatiramer Acetate, an immune modulator. It has proven some effect in the animal model of MS, but is yet to be tried in the human model, thus being us. There is still a long way to go to ascertain if this could benefit MS, but is far from a new treatment for MS as advocated by some.

Used in moderation it can certainly only do the body more good than harm, however used in excess amounts you can jeopardise your health.   Like any medication it has side effects. These side effects can range from mild to serious that include headache, nervousness, sleep problems, vomiting, diarrhoea, irritability, irregular heartbeat, and tremor, dizziness, ringing in the ears, convulsions, confusion and heartburn. In extreme excess amounts, Green tea can be fatal.

**High Dose Oxygen Therapy (HDOT)** involves breathing through a mask inside a pressurised oxygen chamber. The chamber is actually the same as those used in decompression for divers. A higher than normal concentration of oxygen saturates your blood and tissues. Multiple Sclerosis patients breathe pure oxygen while under increased air pressure in the chamber. Breathing 100% oxygen, and the increase in pressure, results in a higher intake of oxygen in the blood and ultimately in the human tissues. The idea behind this is to repair damage tissue before it becomes scarred. The idea is encourage MS inflammation to heal before it becomes scar tissue. The scar tissue is what ultimately leads to the cut off of the signal from the brain to the limb, preventing impulses from reaching the limb leading to disability.

There are about sixty HDOT Therapy Centres throughout the United Kingdom. The first centre was set up in Dundee in 1983, designing their operations using information from a controlled clinical trial conducted in New York between 1980 and 1982. The treatment is not only for MS but for other conditions like gangrene, strokes and cerebral palsy in children. There are a lot more patient reports that suggest it is beneficial for people with bladder and fatigue problems. During the treatment patients breathe 100% oxygen most of the time to maximise the effectiveness of their treatment, but have periodic breaks during which they breathe room air to minimize the risk of oxygen toxicity. A side effect of this treatment can be blurred vision can be caused by swelling of the lens, which usually resolves in two to four weeks

High Dose Oxygen Therapy anecdotal reports from other countries in the world like USA, Russia, Argentina, Australia and Italy suggest that it helps Multiple Sclerosis Patients.

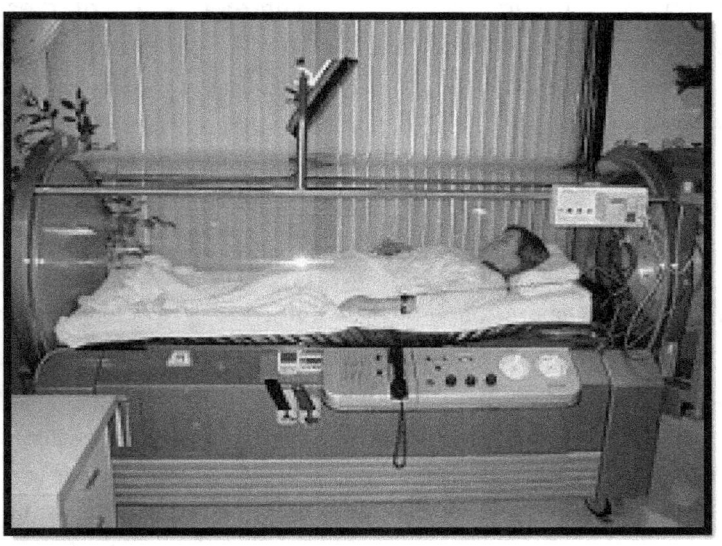

[80] High Dose Oxygen Chamber (Image source: Wikipedia. Author: James Heilman, MD)

A Recent study analysis of this evidence suggests there is no clinically significant benefit from the administration of HDOT. The great majority of randomized trials investigated a course of 20 treatments at different pressures daily for 60-120 min over 4 weeks against a placebo group. No significant benefit of HDOT on the clinical course of MS was identified in this review. It remains possible that HDOT is effective in a subgroup of individuals not clearly identified in the trials at that stage, but in any event, there was no indication of a significant benefit to MS patients.

There may a case for further human trials and for prolonged courses of HDOT at modest pressures, but the case is not strong. At this time, the routine treatment of MS with HDOT is not recommended for Multiple Sclerosis.

Frankly in my opinion, the cost is just not worth the outcome. Until further research is done, I consider this as still yet another money making scheme.

## Vitamins and supplements

There are many vitamins, natural remedies and immune boosters on the market today. Although some of these may be of benefit to you and your Multiple Sclerosis, these are limited to a handful. And just as the amount of herbal remedies and vitamins, the amount of "pushers" is high. The internet is full of these "peddlers'" web pages and the advantages for you. The ultimate reality is very few of these will stand the rigors of testing in trials and FDA regulations. However, I am not going to shoot these down outright, as many of these have a benefit to you whether you have MS or are a normally healthy person. However, get these from a health store or drug stores from people with the right knowledge, and also notify your doctor of what alternative vitamins etc. you do take.

The internet pedlars will add studies that have never even being verified or proven in a lab with the right credentials. There are literally thousands of warning letters from the FDA to these companies and "peddlers'". Be careful with these choices out there, and do background checks on these by the FDA (there website www.fda.gov is a good place to start) or other medical watchdogs. Avoid any supplement or natural remedy that claims it can boost the immune systems. We, as MS patients, need to down regulate the immune system not boost it.

## A Vitamin D supplement: is it good for Multiple Sclerosis?

The lack of correct levels of Vitamin D has long been suggested as a possible factor in developing Multiple Sclerosis. The only way to get enough vitamin D is through exposure to sunlight and through diet, but there may be times when you need to consider supplementing to attain the correct levels of Vitamin D. This is certainly the case if you cannot get outside sunlight exposure.

The groups of people that are advised to take vitamin D supplements include:

- Women who are pregnant or breastfeeding.

- People over 65.

- Those exposed to incorrect levels of Vitamin D under the age of 18.

Vitamin D is currently under study as a supplement to treat Multiple Sclerosis attacks or flare up, however initial indicators are it may be beneficial to speed up recovery time by a very small margin. However, Vitamin D and especially high levels thereof, is not recommended as a so-called standalone treatment of a flare up. This is advocated by some groups, and these include the so called "Supplement Peddlers". There is no conclusive study that indicates Vitamin D as a treatment for MS. But there are studies that indicate maintaining the correct levels of Vitamin D can reduce the number of relapses, even if it only a small percentage value for you.

"There's mounting evidence that low vitamin D levels influence the disease" says Andrew Solomon, who specializes in treating MS patients.

There is a strong warning that large doses of vitamin D over a long time period can result in toxicity. The signs of toxicity include nausea, vomiting, constipation, poor appetite, weakness and weight loss. Vitamin D toxicity can lead to elevated levels of calcium in your blood, which can result in kidney stones. Always check with your doctor to test for the correct levels and whether a supplement is needed before going to the extreme and risking your health.

This is true with all other forms of supplements and vitamins. These supplements can sometimes have a damming effect in conjunction with your prescribed drugs or disease modifying drugs.

# New Treatments for Multiple sclerosis in the Pipeline

"**ATX-MS-1467** is a therapeutic peptide mixture that will be recognised by at least 70 % of MS patients who have a specific genetic profile. It has been developed by Bristol University spin-off company, Apitope. They believe it could prevent relapses and stop further degeneration as a result of the condition.

ATX-MS-1467 is a new possible peptide therapy that is made up of four short peptides derived from human myelin basic protein. It works by down regulating the immune systems' T-Cell response to myelin basic protein. In plain English, it reduces the immune systems t-cell attack on Myelin, the sheath that protects the nerves in the Central Nervous System. It has a more positive affect as it leaves the immune systems' T-Cell response to other virus or infections intact. In other words, any T-cell that start an immune reaction to Myelin, is down regulated, but any other immune response that protects us from viruses and infection not similar to Myelin will still remain active. This is different from current immune modulating drugs or DMD where the bulk of the immune response is suppressed, making, the body open to opportunistic infections.

The first study was carried out in six SPMS patients, with promising results. This peptide therapy was well tolerated by these MS Patients in the clinical trial with no adverse effects reported during the study. Although the trial was not designed to show efficacy, there was preliminary evidence of a positive clinical response to ATX-MS-1467 in two of the six patients. One patient with Optic Neuritis resulting from the inflammatory process involved in MS continues to demonstrate a clinically significant improvement in visual acuity post treatment. Additionally, a second patient has shown some improvement in the Gadolinium-enhanced MRI scan indicating a reduction in inflammatory processes in the brain.

Apitope, in partnership with Merck Serono, has initiated a second Phase I trial in England and Russia in May 2010. This trial in 40 relapsing MS was designed to evaluate the in this group of patients. The only worry is that this treatment was first announced in 2008, and seems only to go on clinical trials now. A big contributing factor of this treatment going ahead was the partnership between Merck Serono and Apitope. This partnership was in place since 2009 and together with and Fast Forward, LLC, the National Multiple Sclerosis Society's subsidiary devoted in bridging the gap between research and drug development.

The company has reported that the last patient was enrolled in November 2012 but there are no clear indications as to when the results can be expected. However this could lead to the first form of therapeutic halting, and possibly, reversing the damage caused by Multiple Sclerosis."

**Trimesta** is currently being tested on Multiple Sclerosis. Trimesta is being tested as an oral medication that is an immune modulator and anti-inflammatory tablet. The primary ingredient is estriol, which is a hormone. This hormone is produced in the placenta by pregnant women. In short, Estriol is an androgen steroid manufactured by the adrenal glands. Estriol has been on the market for 40 years to treat post-menopausal hot flushes.

Doctors have for a long period noted pregnant woman with relapsing remitting Multiple Sclerosis have had a drastic reduction in their relapses, especially during their third trimester of pregnancy. At this stage their oestrogen levels are at its highest in the pregnancy. There was a sharp drop in the MS symptoms of these pregnant women. Other autoimmune disease symptoms also drastically dropped in this period. Pregnant woman also show a spontaneous remission in the third trimester only to go into a high rate of relapses in the post birth period. Based on the above information, they tested Trimesta in non-pregnant women who have Multiple Sclerosis.

The outcome of these studies has shown a reduction of relapses in a MS patient. There was also a reduction of lesions in MS patients on these trials. MS patients on these trials have also shown an improvement of their cognitive skills on Trimesta. Currently this drug is in a stage three trial. It is still not a cure but could slow down the progress of RRMS in female patients. It is currently only tested on females.

Trimesta is currently in a phase Ii trial, a double-blinded, placebo controlled study of estriol pills versus placebo pills in Relapsing Remitting Multiple Sclerosis. The study treatment will be an added on to Copaxone injections in all subjects. The primary outcome measure is a reduction in relapses. It is a multicentre trial, with 164 patients participating. The outcome of this trial is expected in January 2014.

In January of 2012, Synthetic Biologics, Inc. (Adeona Pharmaceuticals) announced that patient enrolment has been completed in a Phase II clinical trial evaluating the efficacy and safety of oral estriol Trimesta(TM) for the treatment of Relapsing-Remitting Multiple Sclerosis.

**HiCy treatment in Multiple Sclerosis** is currently in clinical trial and stands for High Cyclophosphamide (Cytoxan). Cyclophosphamide is a chemotherapy drug that slows down cell growth and halts it. This drug stops growth of white blood cells but does not stop the reproduction of white blood cells in the bone-marrow. Cytoxan was tested before in normal dosages in Multiple Sclerosis and is still in use as an off label treatment for MS.

With HiCy, treatment they use very high dosages of this drug to stop the body's immune system totally. So they basically wipe out your immune system in one fell swoop. By doing this the, body reproduces white blood cells to regenerate the immune response of the body. This procedure is done to basically "reboot" the immune system. It has shown some promising result in the treatment of MS, but it is not permanent as the immune responses that start the attack on the Central Nervous System will start up again.  This procedure is only done in the worst cases of Multiple Sclerosis where all other treatments failed. Initial results from trails have shown a reduction of 40% EDSS criteria to measure disability. It has also shown an increase in the physical and mental capacity of patient.

HiCy does come with some serious side effect that are normally associated with Chemotherapy, but it leaves you open to a great deal of opportunistic infection as your body's immune response is totally stopped for a while and you will probably catch anything that comes along. HiCy followed by long-term maintenance with glatiramer acetate is well tolerated in patients with MS, and appears to be effective in reducing the risk of relapse, disability progression, and new MRI lesions. Cyclophosphamide is marketed by Baxter International Inc.

There are still a massive amount of new drug treatments and other treatments out there. Since these are still in very early stages of trials and some have major safety concerns attached to it, I feel it is not necessary to write about it now and bring possible false hope to Multiple Sclerosis Patients.

## rHIgM22 anti-body to treat Multiple Sclerosis

rHIgM22 is a new anti-body that is being develop and tested for the re-myelination of the Central Nervous System damage caused by Multiple Sclerosis.

This antibody is a human anti-body that was discovered by the Mayo Clinic. It basically promotes the growth of Myelin, the sheath that covers our nerves. This treatment is being tested on laboratory mice after inducing the Theiler's virus (Bovine virus, found mostly in hoofed animals), that causes mice to develop Myelin loss. After a 5 week treatment of rHIgM22 the Myelin growth was shown in about 83% of the mice. The MRI clearly showed lesion shrinkage in 83% of the mice where Myelin loss was induced with the Theiler's virus.

This anti-body was also tested in mice with spinal injuries and showed very good results. The anti-body was well tolerated by the mice, and no toxic effect was seen, indicating that it can be safely used in humans, as this is a human anti-body.

rHIgM22 was presented to the FDA to start testing in humans soon. If this anti-body does prove to be successful, we may see a new treatment in Multiple Sclerosis in the next couple of years. Further to this, the researchers suggest that this could lead to a vaccine for Multiple Sclerosis by 2020. So there is a lot of hope in the next couple of years.

Human trials are currently being started on rHIgM22. This is a very promising development as it could mean the reversal of the damage caused by Multiple Sclerosis. Acorda Therapeutics and Mayo Clinic announced that 60 patients have been enrolled in the first clinical trial of rHIgM22, a re-myelinating antibody being studied for the treatment of multiple sclerosis. This is a Phase 1 clinical trial enrolling patients with MS to assess the safety and tolerability of rHIgM22.

# Multiple Sclerosis and the effect on your life.

We all start our lives on this "rock" we live on, the "third rock" from the Sun in infancy.  Eventually the majority of us inhabit this planet for the rest of our lives. We all grow up with hopes, dream and expectations of making the best of our brief existence on this "rock". But sadly for a certain amount of humans on this planet, these dreams get shattered and destroyed by no doing of their own. Some at one or other stage get affected by disease and conditions that affect their life and determine their future on this planet.

If you, as a healthy person, have ever looked into the eyes of a young child, whose life is affected by this disease you are overwhelmed by different emotions. They did not deserve it and are innocent little angels living with whatever affects them. But in most cases you will find a supporting and loving family supporting this little angel, as they brave the storms that they fight every day. Parents, grandparents and other family members continue to love and support this little angel, and in most cases complete strangers as well. They are continually supporting this little angel, who faces this world full of uncertainty but with hope and a spirit for living, even if this time on earth for some of them may be very short. There is always a feeling of attachment and involvement by those on the side of these little angels.

However the opposite is always there as well and this is a sad part in human behaviour. Detachment is a very true fact about disease and this also applies to Multiple Sclerosis as well. How many times do we see a Multiple Sclerosis patient sitting on their own in their own little corner in life? They are basically removed from friends and the occasional family member drops by to visit them perhaps once or twice a week. This is a too typical scene that is faced every day, with especially the advanced Multiple Sclerosis patient being left alone in life with nursing services caring for them. But it is also seen in patients that still have some ability in life left in them. Society has either given up on them or they have given up on society. The prospects for these patients dim and they are completely removed from interactions with other persons. Their lives are basically completely void of any meaning or of hope for a future. Added to this, is that certain health structures in governments only provide the bare minimum for these patients. It is a sad result of this disease. Also it does not say much about our actions to fellow human beings. These patients live a life of complete emotional and physical disability. Sadly this reality is also present in all many diseases, but this also is fully avoidable.

During my own life with Multiple Sclerosis I have come into contact with many patients where this plays a very big role in their lives. The hospitals, frail care homes, and other faculties are full of cases like this. The sad fact is we, as humans, do not care about other people's wellbeing; in fact we turn ourselves away of from those persons. Being diagnosed with a debilitating disease like Multiple Sclerosis can for the most of us feel like being a social outcast. Friends are normally the first to detach themselves from this person. It is a phenomenon that we live with every day. The sad fact is these friends are for the most part not informed about what Multiple Sclerosis is and their first reaction is silently, "Can I get infected with this as well". Another question that plays a great roll in this; "What is expected from me to assist my friend?" I think I can answer that question for all of us; "We are only asking for your friendship and expect nothing more from you. Be our friend and do not cut us out of your life, because your friendship means more to us than anything in this world. We did not ask or deliberately went looking for Multiple Sclerosis, it just happened. Learn from us what Multiple Sclerosis is and give us your moral support as this is all we ask."

But the reality of this is it will affect a lot of us. Friends will leave us, as they feel embarrassed to be seen with what appears to others as walking around with the village "drunk". As the disease progresses, this will even get worse. We will stumble and fall, but we will stand up again. Strangers will make rude and nasty remarks about our actions. We will perhaps not be able to keep up with our friends as we go out or go on a shopping trip etc. We may seem lazy to others, but believe me, we are doing the best we can. We may not feel like going out today as our bodies are run down and tired, but bear with us as we have our good days as well. The old friend you knew is still inside our mind and sometimes our bodies. But sadly, only true friends will stay with us, and this physical detachment does take its toll on our friends. This eventually gets worse as we sometimes have to cut loose these ties that bind our friendship, not that we actually want to but we see what effect it takes on you, our friends. So along the way we lose a few friends, sometimes by own choice as we see what effect our Multiple Sclerosis has on our friendship. Our world becomes smaller as our disease progresses and we detach ourselves more from our friends.

This is the very sad reality in life, but real for some Multiple Sclerosis patients. Good family support does go a long way in assisting us in our daily lives. But in certain, if not the majority of cases, this is a very true. In the beginning stages of Multiple Sclerosis we can still rely on good family support, but eventually the disease will take a toll on this as well. Families stop inviting you over to gatherings as they fear you may embarrass them in front of their friends. Having a glass or two of wine may end up portraying you as the "town drunk". Some family members will try to avoid you as they do not know how to present you to the world out there. In certain cases, they have not fully acquainted them with what Multiple Sclerosis actually is, and true, in certain case they are afraid of what to expect from this new development in your life. Disease always has a stigma attached to it, and is always in the back of someone's mind, perceived to be contagious. I think most of you have heard the following at one stage in your life;" Is it contagious?" No matter how hard you explain this fact, a few will not be very convinced of it. This is also true of friends too, and that can also explain their detachment from you.

The worst scenario is the fact that we, as Multiple Sclerosis patients, are at one or other stage reliant on family support in life. But eventually this will become a problem to them as well. Not all families are emotional and physical adept to deal with this issue and this is true even of some spouses as well. Eventually, this will take its toll on them. Dealing with a sick child is a total different scenario than dealing with a sick adult. Multiple Sclerosis has taken a toll on many a marriage that was not strong enough to survive it. Even in strong marriages, the feeling of detachment tends to arise. Some are strong enough to survive this, but experience has taught me that this can be a very bumpy road with many failings along the way. I have seen this not only in my own life but in other lives as well. Once the family support dwindles, a feeling of detachment develops in Multiple Sclerosis patients, and we tend to withdraw more and more from society. Certain patients feel like they have become a burden on society and their families and eventually the patient give up on life itself. A certain feeling of detachment starts to develop. This eventually leads to emotional and physiological detachments adding to a mountain of problems that are already there. It comes to a point where we detach ourselves from this world, and eventually this leads to a cascade of events that will only worsen instead of helping us on this difficult path that we walk.

I know I paint a grim picture, but we need to face these facts. This could ultimately lead to detachment from family friends and the world if we are not careful. This is probably the biggest reason why certain patients are rather shipped off to frail care homes, as families are scared about the disease or do not know how to handle a person with Multiple Sclerosis. Multiple Sclerosis patients tend to get lost in this system and forgotten about. This eventually has a devastating effect on the patient itself and they detach from this world. They become a prisoner within themselves, trapped in a body, they did not choose, and eventually give up on life. But we have the power to change our destiny.

From the very beginning of your diagnosis of Multiple Sclerosis, arm yourselves with all the knowledge out there, so that you can become a light for family and friends to follow. After all we did not choose the disease, nor inflicted it on ourselves. It chose us. Educate your friends and family about what to expect from you, and what you expect in return. We actually do not need your sympathy so much, but we need your emotional support and understanding about the disease. Learn from us about what we can and cannot do. Bear with us in days that we are not feeling able to enjoy life to the fullest; we are limited some days in what we can do. Don't cut us out, we are still us, but we have a few more problems to deal with. Lift us up when we need it, but do not pity us. Help us to educate others about this disease. Help us become a light for others to follow, and assist us in our cause to help ourselves and others. Criticise us when we need it, we are stronger than what you think. When we fall, don't hold us down, but allow us to stand up and fight another day. Positive actions lead to positive outcomes in our lives. Care about us as we would care about you if this had happened to you under the same circumstances.

The important thing to remember here is to avoid detachment from life itself. Join a support group, as your actions together will inspire and electrify others around you. Be a fighter, not a retreater. Don't let negativity get you down, fight back with positivity. Get involved in your own treatment, ask questions and get answers. Know what you can do and inform others about your limitations. Schedule your life around your abilities and let your friends know about this. This will lead to a better understanding about you. But do not detach yourself from this world, as you have as much right as any able person to live on this "rock".

## The Effect of Multiple Sclerosis in my life.

There is an old saying that goes; "Preacher practice what you preach".

I must say through my life I have been guilty of not heeding my own preaching's, and I have allowed Multiple Sclerosis to get the better of me, and this cost me greatly in my life. I have given up hope at stages in my life. Yet today I stand back and look where I came from and knowing exactly where I am going. Some, if not all, set out in this chapter was true in my case, and is still playing a huge part in my life. I needed to look back on my life to see where I went wrong. What follows is a brief overview of my life.

Back in 1984 I got married for the first time, and we were both free spirited persons with a rebel inside both of us. Our son was also born out of this relationship. We were young and we were wild. Marriage was not intended for us and we split a couple of years later. It was a roller coaster ride and we eventually got back together and spent the next couple of years together. Back in those years, my wife had an uncle who had Multiple Sclerosis and little did we know that this would also affect us one day.

Through all my trouble and eventually my diagnosis, my first wife was there for me all the way. In 1993 I was diagnosed with Multiple Sclerosis, although I could not trace it to a family member in my direct ancestral line. I had lost my job in that year, and also tended to believe that chemicals in my work environment accounted for my disease. I was in the office printing equipment industry for the most part of the 1983 until 1991, and I also lent my ears out to others that my MS was caused by the strong chemicals we were exposed to.

I spent a couple of months recuperating from my first attack and was also on a six month interferon drug trial. The trial ended and slowly but surely I got better on my own. I changed direction in life and went into the building industry. For the next years I had no difficulty and did not suffer any relapses for the 4 years. But a big surprise was waiting for me.

During the first three years of our marriage, my first wife had two episodes of Phlebitis and this was not contributed to any disease. She visited the emergency room twice for severe redness of the eyes and inflammation in the eye. Her one eye was blood shot and red, and she was given medication for it. Little did we know that inside her body, there was a silent disease inside her brain. In 1997 she suffered from severe tremors and numbness in her legs. And that year she was diagnosed with Multiple Sclerosis. This was the biggest shock of my life and hers. We could trace her MS back to her direct ancestor, but not mine. The doctors were also a bit baffled by this. There were lots of question but no answers. Nowhere in the history of Multiple Sclerosis was there any indication that this disease is contagious, and this is still the case today.

I suffered a minor relapse in 1998 but got over this one soon. But MS had claimed a victim and four years later our ways parted for good. I could very well deny that Multiple Sclerosis had a role to play in it, but I would be lying. It played a significant role in the regression of our union. Today I can say with certainty that MS: Multiple Sclerosis played a big role in our parting. Our marriage was not built on a firm foundation, but rather on shaky ground. My Multiple Sclerosis did not impact on my life as severely as MS has impacted on hers. Our biggest concerns were for our son as well. Having one parent with MS is bad enough, but with both of us afflicted by this, his chance of developing MS is surely far greater today. Thankfully today, at the age of 27, he has not shown any signs of Multiple Sclerosis and we can only hope that this will continue to be the case. My first marriage ended a short while later and we parted as friends.

By the end of 2004 I was involved in a relationship and was busy with a construction job. The company that I was working for however declared bankruptcy and my life took a turn for the worse. We also discovered that my partner was pregnant. The first thing that popped into her mind was, if this unborn child could also develop Multiple Sclerosis. I can still today recall the discussion in my parents' house, as we were living in a flat behind the house. Knowing the history of my first marriage, one of her concerns was whether she also could be infected by this disease, and what about our baby. It took some convincing that there was no risk to her, but there could be very small risk that our child might be one day affected by MS.

By January 2005 I was under a lot of strain, as we had a child on the way and we were flat broke and the future looked dark. This caused my Multiple Sclerosis to act up a bit. I was drained of energy and the slightest touch would cause a pain on my right side of my face. Another symptom at that stage was typical sensory ataxia.

My hands and feet had a continuous burning sensation, and the slightest touch would exacerbate this. Silently I knew I was in relapse, not severe but strong enough to affect my life and my relationship. I would shy away from affection from my partner as I did not want to tell her what was going on. A roller-coaster of emotion was running inside me. I knew if I told her she would have taken her sisters advice and aborted the baby, and that was the last thing I wanted.

I bit the bullet, and tried to be as strong as I could. By May of that year I gained employment in the building industry again. The construction industry involved some hard work and being in the sun the whole day certainly did not help me, but I had to carry on. I was walking with a continuous limp and blamed it on a fall on site, but deep inside I knew the truth. About two month after our daughter was born; life started changing again for me. I gained new employment as a project manager, although it was more challenging to the mind, the physical activity was far less. This led to a major change in my Multiple Sclerosis, the nagging symptoms started disappearing again, on their own, and being more financially sound, my stress levels dropped way down.

By end 2005 I was well enough again and we enjoyed life as a couple and in March 2006 we got married. For next 18 months all was fine in our lives, we enjoyed living, spending time together and we seemed blissfully happy. By end 2006 I heard the shocking news that my employer had terminal cancer, and his business would not survive after his death. Again I had to my make choices, and it was probably the wrong choice, but the financial incentives were lucrative at the time. I took a job as a hands-on supervisor knowing full well that I might jeopardise my health again. The job started in January of 2007 and with that two of the hottest month in that year.

By end February 2007 my silent enemy was back in full force again, and sent me to the emergency room on many occasions. May month came and it was confirmed I have Multiple Sclerosis and was in active relapse. This was my worst year of my life, but luckily I had some savings built up and financially I could survive. As far as employment, there was a big hole which I was out in again. I decided to take some consultancy work just to keep the boat afloat. But I noticed that somehow my wife became distant, and this worried me. We had some tough times financially, but we got by. There was enough money to survive but none for extravagances and the medical bills were piling up.

In August of that year, I teamed up with a partner, and together we built a 5 story structure. Financially we were sound, but I still had nagging MS symptoms with the occasional flare up. The construction project was physically demanding, and did take a toll on my life. Steroids about three times a year kept me going. I was not in any financial position to afford disease modifying drugs. By the end of 2008 we completed the project, but this was the time of a great slump in the building industry and work was few and far between and luckily I landed a project doing a pipeline.

This project was very demanding and I suffered a lot of major setbacks with my MS but carried on working, even though I was declared medically unable to do physical work. This put a severe strain on me, but I had to carry on. MY EDSS was scored at 5 and I knew that I was in a very bad situation. I was suffering from major fatigue as well. I noticed the strain in my married life and decided to carry on despite my condition. By January 2010 my employers noticed that I was taking major strain, and decided to reduce my time on site. This helped a bit, but I was under continual MS attack, to the extent that it border lined on primary progressive MS. Eventually in May, I was retrenched as the company was not doing well and downsized. I continued to work until June on a consultancy basis only. This is when I decided to learn more from this enemy called MS

My wife, by then had become a stranger to me. She distanced herself from my MS and me, and even went so far as calling my "MS hugs" as attention seeking, and her family even suggested that as well. This, I would learn later in my divorce papers. I was even accused of bluffing having MS, and was called too lazy to work. Although at that stage, I was hoping that this would pass and we could be a family. Noticeably, help from her family was few and far between and they even distanced themselves from me. My own family were too far away to help.

By end July, I was financially drained, and in a desperate attempt to salvage my marriage with my wife, whom I still dearly loved back then, I decided to get some rest from it all. We had no money and soon would have no place to stay. We sold most of our belongings, and this was a joint decision to move back to my parents, hoping for a bit of a rest and a fresh start. We left with what we could and even had to leave some belongings behind. Of course, on requesting her family to help us get our possessions out of the place, none responded. In another desperate attempt, I decided to give the rest away. The vultures came out and within a half an hour her family took whatever they could lay their hands on, for the next couple of days.

During the next six months I still suffered from setbacks, but we were in safe hands and it looked like my marriage might survive, even though my wife was still distant to me. I needed steroids as well, but our government hospitals, in that area where my parents stayed, were unable to give it. Again I weathered the storm, talking plenty of rest and slowly building my strength back. By December, we were offered an opportunity by my wife's other family to move in with them in a different town, with the promise of starting a company together. My wife and I grabbed this opportunity with both hands as my parents were living in a small town back then, whose main income was tourism; there were few opportunities to make money. Added to the fact, the primary caregivers were not financially able to provide for all our needs.

So we set sail to my sister-in-laws place with great promises of going into business together. I was still in on-going relapse but the opportunity sounded great. This was the worst disaster of my life. I realised that in the first two weeks, but kept my mouth shut. The first promise of me getting a bus ticket back down to attend my son's wedding did not materialise. Until this day I am still unable to forgive myself for that. We did, however, try to start a company, but with little or no financial support from my in-laws. I realised I was in this for the long haul on my own. I, too, soon realised that my sister in-law needed a play mate and shopping partner while her husband was working in Africa.

Now the one thing that I knew, was that if I was ever going to get well again I needed to relax, and take breaks whenever needed, and this I did do. If only I knew what the consequences of that would be. By this time, I was caught up into something I did not want to be in. Yet I powered on parking myself in front of my laptop and doing web pages and so forth. We started a business listing site as well, and my wife lent a hand there, but the constant interruptions of going to do shopping with the sister in law, made this nearly an impossible task to achieve on my own. During the weekends there was constant drinking going on, with myself abstaining from this as I am not a drinker.

Silently I suffered my MS attacks as I would have neither sympathetic an ear to lean on nor the financial ability to get a steroid treatment when needed.  I needed help to get this business started but the help that I got was next to nothing. Another complication would be diet wise, while the wife and sister in law, on their nearly now daily shopping sprees would eat food somewhere; I was by now slowly starving. All I could pray for was a miracle. However with the decline in my diet, plus lack of medication, I was getting worse. A simple task like making coffee was to me a mountain to climb. Walking to the bedroom to get pills would literally drain all my energy.

By July, my sister in law started speaking to me in an aggressive manner, but I had to suck it up. I had no place to go. I knew I needed out. I just had to get out of there, for my daughter's sake as well. As a family, my wife also wanted to move away from there. Eventually in October of 2011, we moved to a farm where the rent was cheap. I could barely afford it, but it was like heaven to me. I was on my own with my family, and hope that my shaking marriage would survive. My wife expressed her joy in the new place, and many of my neighbours and friends will testify to that in court. In January 2012 business was still slow but we were scrapping along by the skin of our pants. But I still noticed a cold distant feeling from my wife.

The same manner that was evident at my sister-in-laws house was also presenting it self here. It would be a constant battle getting her up in the mornings to help me with the business. My recovery was slow, but I was getting there. On the occasions that we did visit my sister in-law or they visited here, I was pushed aside and my feelings about my wife's liquor consumption was ignored.  Another factor playing a major role in our marriage is the complete breakdown of our sex life. I could not afford the smart pills for the "soldier" and it was evident that our intimate moments were far and few apart. From my part, the lack of the correct medication and to a certain extent, my libido levels were way down. From her side, it was the total lack of interest in our sex lives, with her knocking herself out at night with my painkillers and prescription schedule 5 medication.

Then in July, the bomb burst. I noticed that there were very little input from my wife's side in the business, and she was sleeping late every morning, and using my pain killers to knock herself out every night. It was only then that I realised that she was busy talking to men on Social Media Pages and even flirted with them, then actually helping me in the business. By now, I knew that my marriage was doomed. Confronting her, she walked out and moved back in with her sister-in-law. Only then also did I also realise that my daughter was in danger living there. For legal reasons I cannot divulge the nature of these dangers. My business was just about in the gutter, also a result of her neglecting her responsibilities and functions in the business.

A Couple of weeks later, when I approached the children's' advocate and an attorney on how to keep my daughter safe, they advised me I can just keep her, if it is for her safety. Two days later my wife arrived with the police to remove my daughter. They eventually left empty handed as my daughter wanted to stay with me. Out of pure spite, they left me stranded high and dry by taking my vehicle away, which was registered in her name, yet she can't even drive. Luckily my neighbour lent me one of his vehicles.

The next morning she applied for a family violence protection order, but this was not successful. The very next night I had another visit from the police to take my daughter, but yet again they left empty handed as my daughter wanted to stay. This happened after I invited her to visit her child. Out of kindness, I set up a temporary parental plan on a week by week basis, of which the terms was broken by her in the first week. Being kind and not wanting to let my daughter be without her mother I let her stay over with her again. Only to be back stabbed by her taking my child 1400km away from me; an hour after she picked her up.

Then the divorce papers came. I was utterly shocked by the allegations in them. Going through them, I realised that a much gloomed picture was painted of me. I was called lazy, did not want to work, knowing full well I was declared medically unfit to work. According to them, my brother in law organised construction jobs for me and I did not take them. (Although the exact opposite is true, I organised sub contract work for him when he was retrenched.) She also refuted the fact that I did have MS and portrayed me as a person that did not want to work. She denied the fact that she knew about my Multiple Sclerosis, even though it was discussed with her in front of witnesses.

I was called a sponger, even though the only record of a loan to me was about $500 for the business. I was accused of being controlling and asking for coffee every half an hour, even though we could hardly afford coffee at that stage. Asking for lunch was a fruitless task, and my daughter and I started eating dry bread for lunch, as she was always in front of her computer on Social Media Pages.

I was accused of using massive amounts of pills, even though they were prescription drugs, and far from what I actually needed, as I could not afford the drugs that I needed. I was on the cheapest drug to control spasms and some neuropathic pain. The pain killers were over the counter drugs, and yes I might have used 2 a day more than the advised dosage, I could not afford the stronger stuff suggested. And to top it all, she consumed some of these every night to knock herself out, and even at times my prescription drugs, leaving me to ponder why I am short.

The most outrages claim, was that these drugs caused violent mood swings. Taking into account this was a mild sedative and sleeping pills, and none of their side effects were violent mood swings. The pain killer's side effects are drowsiness. Somewhere along the line they pick up mood swing in other MS meds and decided to throw this in as another reason for a divorce. And even went so far as to get another protection order against me, with both of them failing in court. My ability to be a father to my daughter is also called into question as I have Multiple Sclerosis.

It was only after she moved out that I would realise the real reason behind her actions. Her sister-in-law was moving back to another town, and the very thought of her living with a "Poor Cripple", as she so eloquently put it one day, scared her. I also found out, that this moving out, was planned by her and her sister, because I have MS and have trouble earning a decent income.  I do earn a liveable wage and can provide for a family, but the luxuries will have to stand aside for now. Never once did she offer to go out and work, but in the divorce she claimed that I refused to let her work. In the good times she suggested that she go and work, but as it was not necessary as we were living more than comfortably. We agreed then that she would rather stay at home and raise our daughter. Strangely though within a couple of days after securing a job, she left it all and ran off with my child.

What struck me most was that anyone could be so cruel as to set their own feelings in front of family. I am shocked and appalled that any person can do this to someone who has only been kind to them. I took her son in as my own and raised him, after he was shunted around from one relationship to another. I am deeply saddened by the fact that she knew the potential danger to my daughter yet chose to live a life of liquor and partying above her own child's safety. However I am deeply shocked by the fact that there are persons out there, supposed loved ones, that will use your disease against you in a divorce to cover their own mistakes and lies.

But it is my genuine belief that eventually the court will see right from wrong, and restore my parental rights with full parental duties. It is clear as daylight that she told lies under oath in her protections orders, of which there are now two of them, that were not granted. The one differs completely from the other and also the fact that there is a clear record and witnesses that will indicate that I have never been violent to her nor spoken hard words to her in my life. To this her son, my stepson, will testify too. I have evidence to back all my claims, and she, by her own words will trip up in court.

I guess that sums up about my life so far, and yes I have lost all that I loved, however not all that loved me. I am now convinced that I was never really loved by my wife, but rather used by her to live a good life. Even though I loved her at one stage; I have lost all respect and feelings for her in the last six months. I am of the firm belief that she did not see her way forward with a "crippled and a poor" husband who has Multiple Sclerosis. As to the meaning of for better or worse etc. only the first part of each counted.

During the last six month I am now practicing what I preach. I will not let this get me down any more, nor am I going to let it influence my life further complicating my Multiple Sclerosis. I have lost 20kg in the last two years, seriously damaging my health, but I am slowly gaining that back. I am for the first time, actually getting over my relapses, and hopefully I can remain relapse free for the next couple of years. I am more active than before, and eating correctly. This has set me on a path to a new and better life. The problem that I am having with custody etc. is temporarily and soon my financial position will all change for the better. I am not going to let this get me down. My day will come when I will triumph above these problems.

Also my message to you, in the last years I have come across many cases of separations and divorces over MS, and believe me, if they do not want to stand with you when you are at your low point, they are not worthy of you at all. Those who do not accept you are in the gutter, so to speak and are not worthy of your affection. Only strong marriages will survive MS and all its flaws. Those that pick you up when you fall, support you when you stumble are the ones that deserve you. The marriages without strong foundation and love will falter. It begs the question; "Do I really need such a marriage?"

For that hopeless fool that leaves you in your time of need, will do it to others as well. Shame and guilt will follow them for the rest of their lives and they will never find internal peace. You pick the fruits of what you sow, and one day these fools will have to eat those rotten fruits themself. I will go to my grave knowing that I made the right choices in life, be it maybe not the right people, but I tried to make the best of it. And one day, if I do not get custody of my daughter, she will read this and understand what her father chose. I will live my life to the fullest, no matter what gets thrown to me by Multiple Sclerosis or fools in my life.

Live your life on the planet called earth, "the third rock from the sun", and bask in its glory and beauty. Don't give up on life; it is the only one you have. Don't become the prisoner within, but set yourself free. We live only but once, but we are still alive and kicking, be it with a bit more difficulty. Don't give up on your hopes, dreams and expectations but adapt them to suit you. Live your life!!!!!!!!!!

# Epilogue

Hope: the dictionary describes it as follows "a feeling that something desirable is likely to happen". The Latin word for this is "spero". Well we all who have Multiple Sclerosis had this feeling at one stage in our lives and to certain extent more than once. This small little word that consists of four letters has had far more meaning than any other word in the whole dictionary. "Hope" is also my message to you.

I remember the first time when I was diagnosed, this word came into play. I knew that there was a likelihood that it was MS but I also had the "hope" that it may not be Multiple Sclerosis. But the diagnosis was confirmed and the meaning of this small word took on a new meaning in my world. The day after my diagnosis I still remember thinking that the doctor telling me that as yet there was no cure, he did give me "hope" that one day this cure will be found as they are doing ground breaking work in the field of medicine.

Living in a country, where we are about 5 years on average behind any other modern country in the world; I looked back into history and remembered Louis Washkansky. Today that name has long been forgotten in history, but it meant something to me. He was the first person ever in the world to receive a heart transplant, but even better, this was done here in my country, just about 10 miles from where I received my diagnosis. This gave me hope that if we were able to do this here, we might be able to find a cure for this disease that I have. My hopes were even more uplifted when I received a phone call a couple of weeks later asking me if I wanted to partake in a drug trial that could benefit me.

I had no idea what I was getting in and how safe this all was, but I now had "hope". It was explained to me that this new drug, an Interferon could at least slow down this disease. I was frightened because in those years all I knew about Multiple Sclerosis was it could put me in a wheelchair, be it in the short term or in about 10-15 years. But my fears were even worse as I had lost my vision for a period, and this could happen any day again with very little warning. My emotional and my logical thinking were in conflict with each other. My heart telling me; Take this drug", but my mind was telling me; "What if it does me more harm than good". Eventually I signed on the dotted line accepting the fact if it does not help me or even harm me, I am in the fortunate position to contribute to science and help others in the future. The trail ran its course and I still had relapses, and my "hope" was a bit dashed.

Eventually over time, I accepted my fate, but a new "hope" was looming. I started getting better on my own, and the number and intensity of relapses decreased and eventually stopped. For about four years I was, what I thought Multiple Sclerosis free and my "hope" for a better life was there as well. The next MRI confirmed this and the only long term reminder being the one constant lesion in the vision centre. In the back of my mind was still that slight caution from the doctors that it could return one day. But still I had "hope" as time was on my side, and perhaps "I hoped" with the next round there will be better medication and also a cure. With a very few problems over the next couple of years I was leading a productive life again, but most of all I had "hope". And even though my Multiple Sclerosis returned again in 2006 with a vengeance, I still turned my head to science and medicine for that "hope".

I guess this is about the point where I have to get my message through in this story, before I bore the pants off you all. We are faced with new challenges each day in Multiple Sclerosis, but we are also faced with new "hope" every day. Even a trial on a new medicine or procedure, no matter how big of a disappointment it may turn out to be, still gives us "hope". Now this is where I can see the reaction on all your faces, how does a failed trial give us "hope"? Multiple sclerosis is a disease of mystery and also a big puzzle consisting of pieces that may or may not fit. With every bit of this puzzle that we prove does not fit we are that much closer to get the pieces that do fit. So, in a sense, with every mystery that we exclude, we are one step closer to finding a cure. And that gives us "hope" that we will cure this disease one day. But the biggest "HOPE" is that of trials on medicine, and procedures that may put us closer to a cure or even a stop in progression.

Never give up "hope", take this four letters with you on your journey through life.

**"Dum spiro, spero , "While I breath, I hope""**

# Copyright Information

www.ingramcontent.com/pod-product-compliance
Lightning Source LLC
Chambersburg PA
CBHW070855290526
45795CB00001B/136